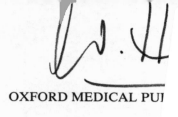

OXFORD MEDICAL PUBLICATIONS

Hip replacement

THE FACTS

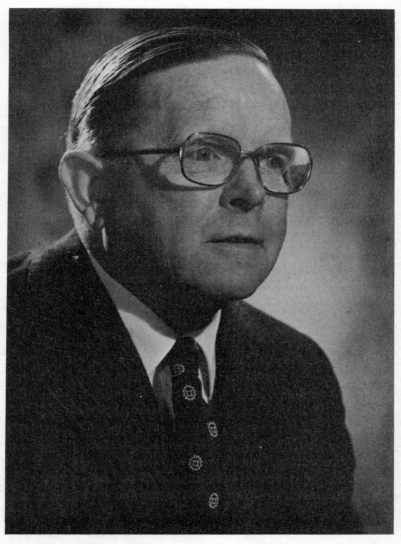

Sir John Charnley (1911–82).

Hip replacement

THE FACTS

with chapters on other joint replacements

KEVIN HARDINGE
M.C.G.O.H. FRCS
M.Ch.Orth.

*Consultant Orthopaedic Surgeon, Wrightington Hospital, Appley Bridge,
Lancashire; Honorary Clinical Lecturer in Orthopaedics, University of
Manchester; Hunterian Professor, Royal College of Surgeons of England*

Illustrations by Joan Taylor

OXFORD NEW YORK TORONTO
OXFORD UNIVERSITY PRESS
1983

Oxford University Press, Walton Street, Oxford OX2 6DP
London Glasgow New York Toronto
Delhi Bombay Calcutta Madras Karachi
Kuala Lumpur Singapore Hong Kong Tokyo
Nairobi Dar es Salaam Cape Town
Melbourne Auckland
and associates in
Beirut Berlin Ibadan Mexico City Nicosia

OXFORD is a trade mark of Oxford University Press

British Library Cataloguing in Publication Data
Hardinge, Kevin
Hip replacement.—(Oxford medical publications)
1. Artificial hip joints
I. Title
617'.581   RD549
ISBN 0-19-261393-6

Library of Congress Cataloguing in Publication Data
Hardinge, Kevin.
Hip replacement, the facts.
(Oxford medical publications)
Bibliography: p.
Includes index.
1. Artificial hip joint—Addresses, essays, lectures.
2. Arthroplasty—Addresses, essays, lectures. I. Title.
II. Series.
RD549.H37   1983   617'.581'0592   83-11483
ISBN 0-19-261393-6

Set by Colset Private Ltd Singapore
Printed in Great Britain by R. Clay & Co.,
Bungay, Suffolk

To

Sir John Charnley, CBE, FRS, FRCS
(1911–82)

All royalties from the sale of this book are to be donated to the Wrightington Hospital Education Centre Trust for the purpose of building the John Charnley Education Centre, Wrightington Hospital, Appley Bridge, Lancashire, for research into and dissemination of knowledge of total joint replacement and rheumatological disorders to medical and paramedical disciplines and patients.

Preface

The 'plastic' hip operation is now an accepted part of our life-style. If you have a 'worn out' hip you can have it replaced in just the same way as if you have a sore throat you can ask your physician for some penicillin tablets. There are reasonable parallels between the discovery of penicillin and the development of the plastic hip.

Alexander Fleming, working in the pathology laboratory at St Mary's Hospital, Paddington, London, in 1928 observed that colonies of *Staphylococcus areus* (the pus-producing bacterium) failed to grow in those areas of a culture that had been accidentally contaminated by the green mould *Peni cillium notatum*. After isolating the mould he found that it produced a substance capable of killing many of the common bacteria that infect man and he called this substance penicillin.

The contamination of the culture plates had probably occurred by mould blowing in through the open window of the laboratory and no doubt this event had occurred before many times all over the world, but the people who had previously observed such spoiled cultures probably regarded them as contaminated plates fit only to be discarded as soon as possible. Alexander Fleming, however, seeing this seemingly everyday event, realized its significance and thus initiated the golden age of chemotherapy whereby the fear and desolation created by infective diseases was markedly reduced.

In a similar way, the plastic hip operation came about from the observation by John Charnley that the fundamental fault with degenerative joint disease and the accepted joint replacement of the day was due to a breakdown of lubrication.

The story that a 'squeak' should lead to the eventual relief of pain to literally millions of people suffering from hip arthritis is worth the telling and it will be of interest not only to those 250 000 people in Europe and North America who undergo the operation annually, but also to others who are interested in what now constitutes an essential part of modern living.

The explosion in the work on total joint replacement that has evolved from the work of John Charnley has not only made orthopaedic surgery the biggest and most rapidly expanding branch of surgery but has also created a multi-million dollar industry on both sides of the Atlantic and has resulted in the formation of new disciplines in universities for the study of the behaviour of materials in the body and the design of implants to replace bones and joints — these new disciplines form a cross-over between biology and engineering, and come under the generic name 'bio-engineering.'

As a result of these advances in medical technology more can now be done for the patient, but the consultation in the doctor's office may not tell the patient everything he wants to know about his condition and its treatment.

In this book, I shall try not only to explain the condition of degenerative joint disease and the operations to replace the diseased joints but also to show how the present level of practice has been reached and how the patient can make the most of his new joint.

Wrightington Hospital is 50 years old in 1983. As a result of the work of Sir John Charnley it has become one of the most famous orthopaedic hospitals in the world.

Wrightington   K.H.
March 1983

Contents

1

What is arthritis and how is it caused?

The joints of the human body are masterpieces of engineering, moving easily and with very little friction between the moving parts.

The two bones that form a joint (Fig. 1) are capped with cartilage, a sort of elastic gristly material. A thin membrane called 'synovium' forms a pouch around the joint and the joint capsule lies outside the synovium and holds the bone ends together. Muscle tendons attached near to the bone ends produce movement of the joint. Finally, around the joints, pockets of fluid (or bursae) lie under the tendons to ensure the smooth movement of these tendons over the underlying bone.

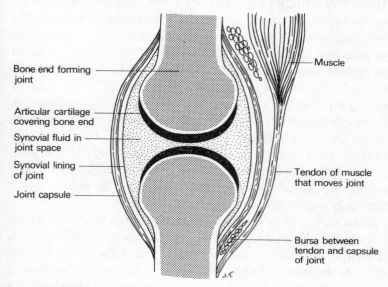

Bone end forming joint

Articular cartilage covering bone end

Synovial fluid in joint space

Synovial lining of joint

Joint capsule

Muscle

Tendon of muscle that moves joint

Bursa between tendon and capsule of joint

Fig. 1. A normal joint.

Hip replacement: the facts

The bones of the joint normally move together without much friction because the cartilage round the bone ends is very shiny and smooth. However, under the microscope, the surface of the cartilage can be seen to be pimply like an orange skin, with numerous lumps and pits. The synovium produces a lubricant which percolates throughout these pits in the cartilage, and when we walk this lubricant is squeezed out over the surface, rather like water being squeezed from a sponge.

To work properly the bones in the joint must be properly aligned; the bone ends must be held together; the cartilage must be strong and resilient; the synovium must produce lubricating fluid; and the capsule must support the joint and prevent abnormal movement.

Arthritis means inflammation of the joint. It is not one disease, but a common name for the final result of many degenerative conditions.

Osteoarthritis is a degenerative wear and tear process that affects five million people in the United Kingdom in one form or another, nearly 8 per cent of the population. It is caused by wear and tear. If a joint were never stressed it would not become osteoarthritic. The relatively lightly stressed joints of the upper limbs are less prone to osteoarthritis than the heavily stressed joints of the lower limbs. It is usually an irregularity of the joint that leads to the development of the osteoarthritis, if the irregularity is slight it will be many years before the osteoarthritis develops — the commonest form of hip arthritis after middle age. On the other hand, if the joint surface is disrupted by fracture, osteoarthritis can occur within one to two years of the accident. The skin is never unusually warm over the osteoarthritic joint.

Rheumatoid arthritis is an inflammation of the joints which is not caused by bacteria and which is a chronic condition. It is often accompanied by a mild illness. It usually affects several joints at the same time (polyarthritis). The cause is unknown. It begins with the synovial membrane becoming inflamed and swollen (synovitis). Then much later the synovitis involves the

2

What is arthritis and how is it caused?

cartilage and causes it to become softer and to start wearing away. After a year or two the disease burns itself out but leaves a joint that is permanently damaged. There are one million sufferers in the United Kingdom, including children (juvenile rheumatoid arthritis) and young men and women. Any joint may be affected, but the incidence is higher in the more peripheral joints such as the hands, wrists, knees, feet, and elbows as opposed to the central joints such as the spine, shoulders, and hips. The hips can however be severely affected.

The onset is gradual with increasing pain and swelling due to the synovial thickening. The overlying skin is warmer than normal.

THE CAUSES OF ARTHRITIS

Osteoarthritis of the hip most commonly affects people aged 50–60 years and the disorder comes out of the blue with no easily recognizable cause. It often begins soon after retirement, when the patient may have been looking forward to golf, fishing, or walking. However no one past the age of adolescence is immune; but in younger patients there is usually a clearly recognized cause such as the joint being malformed since birth, Perthes' disease (softening of the head of the thigh bone, of unknown cause) or an old inflammation or injury. In these cases the hip ball or socket is not quite the right shape and the unevenness causes excess rubbing of the lining cartilage so that it wears away. Similarly, *rheumatoid arthritis* can damage the cartilage of the hip and it also affects all age groups.

When osteoarthritis of the hip begins in people of mature years, however, there is usually no obvious cause and we have to look for clues elsewhere. One clue is that hip arthritis is common in West Europeans and is not so common in people living near the Mediterranean. It is not, as you might think, the cold damp climate of Western Europe that causes this difference, since it has been found that osteoarthritis of the

Hip replacement: the facts

hip is just as common among people who have emigrated from cold wet areas in Europe to dry warm climates in Australia, South Africa, and South Western United States as it is among people who have remained at home.

However, hip arthritis does cause more trouble to the patient in cold damp conditions because the capsule of the joint becomes stiffer and it is more painful to move. Just as an athlete warms up his muscles and joint capsules before intense physical activity, so the impaired arthritic joint with a thickened damaged capsule needs to be kept warm and supple if it is to function at all. The reason why West Europeans should be so affected is thought to be evolutionary: for some reason a minor squaring off of the head of the thigh bone (the femur) has evolved, so that the bearing is slightly out of true. This leads to a slow, very gradual wearing down of the cartilage. In a normal joint, the cartilage cells of the lining surface are removed and repaired in the same way as your skin is replaced — but when the surfaces are slightly uneven, the speed of destruction is faster than that of repair, so the cartilage gets worn down.

Some activities can cause uneven joint surfaces in the hip. Fracture dislocations of the hip where the ball and socket joint is broken as a result of severe injury are seen increasingly in young men involved in motor-cycle accidents. Here the joint surfaces are disrupted and, even after excellent treatment, can remain rough so that wear and tear rapidly leads to hip arthritis. This can also occur in a less dramatic way. Ronald Murray and co-workers in the Royal National Orthopaedic Hospital in London followed up groups of men who, as boys, had had varying amounts of athletic activity. The first group had all been pupils at a boarding school where the emphasis was on scholastic achievement rather than games. The second group went to a school in the country where games were not only encouraged but cross-country running was compulsory. It was found in the second group, following them up 30 years later, that there was an increased incidence of degenerative

4

What is arthritis and how is it caused?

change in the hips. These people, probably as a result of excessive activity before their bone ends were fully mature, had damaged the head of the thigh bone and been left with a minor irregularity of the bearing surface which produced arthritis some 30 years later. A further factor in this group was attributed to bowling in cricket. The action usually involves jumping on to the affected leg after delivery (releasing the ball), this producing an excessive strain. This has parallels in baseball where pitching a curved ball involves a snap of the elbow after delivery. As a result of the development of arthritis of the elbow in adult life in these ardent pitchers the curve ball has been banned from Junior League Baseball.

There is no evidence that osteoarthritis is caused by acid in the diet, infection, poison, drugs, food, constipation, or cold and damp, but its effects can be made worse by cold and damp, being overweight, and general lack of fitness.

2

The changes in the joint in arthritis

Arthritis in any joint is a result of wear of the lining cartilage which leads to uncovering of the underlying bone. As the disease progresses, the underlying bone in its turn becomes affected by the arthritic process and loss of the bone substance itself occurs, which leads to shortening of the bone ends. In the hip joint this leads to shortening of the affected leg, but in the knee joint, if the bone loss affects either the inside or outside of the joint predominantly — then bow leg or knock knee is the most noticeable effect.

The hip joint (Fig. 2) consists of the ball formed by the head of the thigh bone (the femur) and the hollow of the hip bone, which forms the socket or acetabulum — so called because it

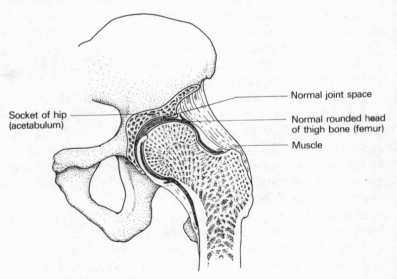

Socket of hip
(acetabulum)

Normal joint space

Normal rounded head
of thigh bone (femur)

Muscle

Fig. 2. A normal hip joint.

The changes in the joint in arthritis

resembles the vinegar cup of Roman times. The head of the thigh bone and the socket are normally covered by extremely smooth and slippery cartilage so that they can easily work and cope with the great loads that are placed on them in normal life.

Ligaments hold these bones together and muscles cause the leverage which results in joint movement. The ball and socket shape of the hip joint permits movement in all directions — forwards, backwards, and side to side — and a combination of all of these movements — rotation. The muscles producing these movements are evenly distributed all around the joint, which is deep seated and surrounded by thick muscles.

If the joint is imperfect, either as a result of a faulty formation at birth (congenital dislocation) or becomes damaged as a result of injury or inflammation, the smooth cartilage gradually becomes worn down and pain and stiffness occur. If the cartilage becomes so worn that bone begins to rub on bone then the joint can lock during walking. This is felt as a grinding vibration and a jarring sensation as the joint comes to a sudden and painful halt. In engineering circles this is known as 'stick slip' when seen in a worn bearing to which extra force must be applied to make it go round. This causes uneven function shown by vibration in the engine.

The loss of leverage in the joint leads to a loss of bulk and power in the muscle and also to a thinning of the shaft of the thigh bone. The thigh bone is a lever on the hip joint, and consists of bony living tissue. If it does less work it thins down. In the fully developed condition, then, the bone end is worn away, there is muscle wasting, and there is thinning of the shaft of the thigh bone.

In osteoarthritis the cartilage of the head of the thigh bone loses its natural resilience and looks dull instead of shiny. It becomes fibrillated — the threads that are interwoven to form the smooth surface become undone and stand on end like a worn carpet, and are gradually shed off. This abnormal wearing away can occur either in normal cartilage which is subjected to abnormal stresses, such as occurs in injuries of the hip joint, or in abnormal cartilage which is subjected to normal stresses.

All cartilage must be supported by the underlying bone — and this bone is a fine meshwork holding the cartilage in place. It is easy to see how severe injury would disrupt this meshwork and cause abnormal stresses. In a similar fashion, however, abnormal cartilage can be produced by micro-fractures of the underlying bone, causing changes in the cartilage, which then becomes unable to withstand normal activity. These minor distortions of the surface of the head of the thigh bone become subjected to repeated minor damage in the course of normal activity. Such repeated minor damage can mount up to produce the same effect as that of a severe injury, leading to osteoarthritis in large weight-bearing joints such as the hip joint and the knee joint.

In these cases there is progressive damage to the cartilage itself. The shiny surface of the cartilage becomes dull, softened, and roughened and small flakes begin to be shed from the surface. Cracks then appear in the cartilage which splits down to the underlying bone, and the bone becomes more dense. As this progresses, the cartilage becomes thinner and eventually wears away, leaving polished bone surfaces articulating with each other. The flakes of cartilage that are shed from the joint surface are absorbed by the synovial membrane lining the joint. This membrane reacts by becoming thicker and producing excessive fluid within the joint, which adds to the discomfort of the patient. At the same time bony spurs (osteophytes) develop around the periphery of the joint.

Thus in the joint which normally has smooth friction-free movement with no sensation, movement becomes limited and painful and rough and grating. Deformities may develop in the form of permanent swelling or deviation of the joint from its normal alignment, in addition to the limitation of range of

The changes in the joint in arthritis

movement and collapse of the joint surface.

The characteristic symptoms are those of pain, initially on movement and use of the joint and later at rest; and swelling caused by fluid within the joint and later caused by the bony spurs around the periphery of the joint. The joint becomes increasingly stiff and deformed. The severity of symptoms will to a large extent depend on the use to which the joint is put once damage is established.

3

Symptoms of degenerative joint disease

PAIN IN THE HIP

The most common symptom of hip arthritis is of course pain and stiffness in and around the hip joint. People vary in their response to pain and sometimes the first symptom they notice is stiffness — they start to have difficulty in cutting their toe-nails, or putting on their stockings. It is remarkable how stiff the hip can become without causing undue pain. The patient may of course just learn to live with the pain. Farmers commonly come up for treatment after having been troubled for many years with extremely stiff hips. They have continued working up to twelve hours a day in spite of having the limp which is caused by wearing away of the joint surface. They have learned to accommodate a gradually deteriorating joint just as they might put up with a creaking gate. On the other hand, a beautician will visit her doctor early to seek treatment for a similar limp, because keeping in good shape is part of her job.

'REFERRED' PAIN IN THE KNEE

The pain is not always localized to the area of the hip joint. The pain from joint wear arising in the hip joint can be partially relieved by drawing the thigh forwards and towards the midline. In the normal circumstances, the foot would be in mid-air and standing and walking impossible. To accommodate this abnormal position the pelvis and spine are tilted to bring the foot down to the ground. This leads to a strain of the other joints involved in weight-bearing while standing or walking. These patients often have pain in the lower back or

10

buttocks, or, more commonly, pain going down the thigh to the knee. There is an aphorism used in teaching medical students 'Pain in the hip, examine the knee; pain in the knee, examine the hip!' These two large joints are supplied by the same nerves and pain arising from one joint may be referred to the other.

It often comes as a surprise to a patient who consults his doctor about a knee pain to be told that the mischief is arising from the hip joint. However, one way of confirming this point is to sit on a table with the thigh fully supported so that the shin is hanging down vertically. In this position it is possible to move the knee and keep the thigh still so that no strain is imparted to the hip joint. If the knee is now kicked straight it is usual to observe that this movement does not cause the sickening pain just above the knee — the pain that is typical of referred pain from the hip.

In about a quarter of people the arthritis affects both hips at once in about equal severity, so that one leg does not become shorter than the other. These patients usually have stiff hips and their walking is changed because the stride length is markedly reduced. They tend to walk more slowly so that the shopping trip that took half an hour some two years previously now takes them over an hour and they feel exhausted afterwards. Stiffness in the hips makes stairs and travel by car difficult. The shortening of the stride length is accompanied by difficulty in moving the feet sideways — so that if sufferers stumble over rough ground or are inadvertently shouldered by someone in a crowd they cannot put their leg to the side to regain balance and often fall down. It is not a loss of balance that leads to this instability, but a loss of ability to regain balance — the result, however, can be the same, a loss of confidence in walking.

MUSCLE WASTING

Walking is produced by considerable leverage around the hip

joint. This leverage depends upon good strong muscles. If the hip joint is worn out, the leverage is reduced and weakening and wasting of the muscles occurs. This muscle wasting can be felt as thinning of the buttocks or thinning of the thigh muscles. The buttock muscles can be checked by placing the hands upon the clenched or tightened buttocks. If one hip only is affected it is easy to detect the difference — if you are one of the unfortunates with two hips simultaneously affected the difference cannot be detected. You may notice however that trousers or skirts that previously fitted well have become baggy and appear too big.

The thinning of the thigh muscles can easily be measured by using a tape measure or simply by looking in the mirror and tightening the muscles, when the difference in bulk can easily be seen.

These muscles become wasted as a result of lack of use. After a successful joint replacement the leverage of the hip joint is restored, but this act alone does not restore the surrounding muscles. Return of muscle power and bulk depends upon a controlled return to full function — the key to which is walking.

PAIN IN THE KNEE

The knee joint (Fig. 3) is a specialized double ball and socket joint where the sockets are like two flat saucers which only partially contain the large double balls. The upper end of the shin bone (tibia) provides the sockets and the lower end of the thigh bone (femur) provides the balls. Situated at the front of the knee joint is the kneecap (patella) which acts as a pulley to allow the quadriceps muscle situated on the front of the thigh to act strongly to straighten the knee joint. When the knee is bent the kneecap glides over the front of the lower end of thigh bone.

The knee joint looked at from the front has a ball and socket on the inside and a further ball and socket on the out-

Symptoms of degenerative joint disease

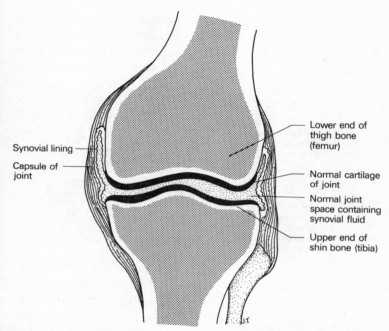

Synovial lining

Capsule of joint

Lower end of thigh bone (femur)

Normal cartilage of joint

Normal joint space containing synovial fluid

Upper end of shin bone (tibia)

Fig. 3. A normal knee joint.

side — called respectively the medial and lateral compartments. When the leg is fully straight, as in standing upright, a small degree of rotation occurs in the knee to lock the joint so that the thigh muscle can relax. From this fully straightened position the knee bends by first rotating to unlock and then gliding and hingeing backwards until the calf touches the back of the thigh. If the weight is off the limb in this position, a great degree of rotation is possible in both directions. The knee joint differs from the hip joint in that it is not near the centre of the body; it is not covered by thick muscle; and it is at the end of the longest lever in the body — the thigh bone. It is thus relatively prone to injury, particularly in active people.

Osteoarthritis and rheumatoid arthritis can both affect the knee joint and lead to severe disability (Fig. 4). Degenerative change can be confined to the joint between the kneecap and

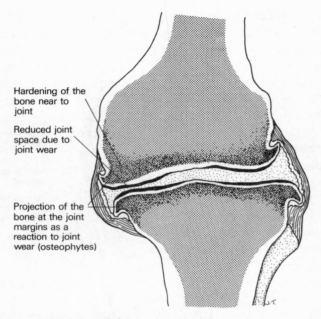

Hardening of the bone near to joint

Reduced joint space due to joint wear

Projection of the bone at the joint margins as a reaction to joint wear (osteophytes)

Fig. 4. An arthritic knee joint.

the thigh bone and here pain is localized to the kneecap and loss of movement is rarely a problem. In the more advanced cases, however, the main joint between the thigh bone and the shin bone is affected with wearing away of the cartilage and this usually spreads to involve the joint of the kneecap and thigh bone as well. The patient notices pain on weight-bearing early on, and has particular difficulty in going up and down stairs. Pain is felt in the middle of the joint, behind the kneecap but can also be felt at the inner and outer side of the joint if either the medial or lateral joint compartment is mainly affected. Fluid accumulating in the joint as a reaction to the joint wear can be a prominent feature and when this causes swelling in the bursa at the back of the knee joint — the so called Baker's cyst — pain can occur in this area.

The pain leads to loss of function and leverage in the joint

Symptoms of degenerative joint disease

with accompanying wasting and weakness of the muscle on the front of the thigh. The wearing away of the articular cartilage means that the normal range of movement is lost. When the knee will no longer bend to a right angle, 90 degrees, going down stairs cannot be performed normally, and the sufferer has to descend one step at a time. When the knee cannot be fully straightened the knee does not lock into its position of stability. On standing the thigh muscle has to remain contracted to hold the knee in this position of strain. This leads to a feeling of weakness in the leg which decreases the functions of both walking and standing.

If the articular cartilage is lost from both the medial and lateral joint compartments equally the overall alignment of the limb remains straight and the main complaint is loss of movement. If articular cartilage and underlying bone is lost either just from the medial or just from the lateral joint compartment, then deformity in the sideways direction will occur. Medial joint compartment damage leads to *bow leg* (genu varum) and lateral joint compartment loss leads to *knock knee* (genu valgum). In the latter case the kneecap tends to drift sideways so that the action of the quadriceps muscle is also displaced sideways and acts like a bow string across the angled joint, this aggravates and increases the knock knee deformity.

It is the specialized ball and socket shape of the knee joint that allows the last deformity that we will discuss here to occur — external rotation leading to *partial dislocation*. Here the muscles and tendons on the outer side of the joint contract and the shin rotates in its long axis so that the foot turns outwards. In the worst degree of this deformity the shin bone moves partially out of joint with the thigh bone so that the edge of the shin bone can be felt as a prominent ridge on the outer aspect of the joint.

Here a distinction must be made between the hip and knee affected by degenerative joint disease. The object of the total joint replacement is to restore as much function as possible.

Hip replacement: the facts

There is rarely urgency in the case of the degenerative hip, in that, from the purely technical point of view, it is possible to get a very satisfactory result even if surgery is carried out after many years of degeneration. In the knee, however, it is unwise to allow gross deformity to occur because it is not always possible to correct and compensate for severe bone loss.

4

Operations for degenerative joint disease

INDICATIONS FOR SURGERY

Total joint replacement is a big operation and involves replacing the joint surfaces. It is primarily carried out where serious destruction of the joint surfaces has taken place. There are other types of operation that are not as extensive and these have a place earlier in treatment of degenerative disease of the hip, knee, shoulder, elbow, wrist, finger, and ankle joint.

1. *Synovectomy*: the surgical removal of the inflamed lining of a joint or tendon sheath.
2. *Debridement*: The 'spring cleaning' of a joint to remove unwanted bony spurs and loose pieces of bone and cartilage floating within a joint cavity.
3. *Osteotomy*: The cutting and re-setting of a bone to re-align a deformed joint.
4. *Arthrodesis*: The fusion of a joint, sometimes known as the 'stiffening operation'.
5. *Arthroplasty*: the repair of a diseased joint to improve its function and reduce or remove the pain.

Synovectomy

The surgical removal of the thickened, inflamed lining of the joint in inflammatory joint disease might be expected to improve symptoms. In practice its benefit and response are very variable. It cannot be proved whether or not the operation prevents further damage to the joint. It is known that this operation relieves pain, but that the synovium may again show the characteristics of the previous inflammatory arthritis. The

17

operation itself can lead to pain and stiffness in the joint.

These complications are prevented by a non-operative synovectomy now being increasingly practised where the joint is injected with radioactive yttrium to suppress the thickened and inflamed joint lining.

Debridement

In a degenerate osteoarthritic joint, pain and disability arise from the presence of bony spurs, roughness of the joint surfaces, and sometimes loose pieces of bone and cartilage which have separated and are floating loose within the joint. Occasionally, therefore, in a suitable joint, which usually means the knee, improvements can be achieved by 'spring cleaning' the joint and removing or smoothing out the irregularities. The results of this operation are variable and difficult to predict because it can never be a precise procedure. The joint surfaces must be fairly extensively damaged for many loose fragments to be formed. This operation will be performed less frequently in the United Kingdom and the United States as the results of total knee replacement are seen to be successful.

Osteotomy

Pain relief and improved function may be achieved by realigning the weight-bearing surfaces of the joint. This is done especially in cases where one part of the joint surface has worn excessively or where deformity (or malalignment) of the joint has occurred. In this way, less worn areas can be brought into use or the deformity corrected. Often when only minor correction of alignment is achieved, pain relief is substantial if the correction reduces the shearing strain on the joint. There is an optimum time for this procedure; deterioration must not have been allowed to go too far. Only certain joints are suitable (knee joints in the early stages) since the joint surfaces must be adequate and relatively intact for the operation to be successful. Osteotomy for osteoarthrosis of the knee is widely practised in the United Kingdom, Europe, and the United States, particularly in younger patients — but is becoming less popular in the elderly because the results are variable and recovery takes a long time.

Arthrodesis

Although one might imagine that stiffening a joint permanently would be disastrous, this is not necessarily true. When only one joint is affected and the joint is producing grave pain and disability, it is often of much greater benefit to the patient to have that joint permanently stiffened so that it is pain-free, stable, and strong, even it if will not bend, than to continue in pain. This has been especially true of wrists and the knees, and even the hip — but the hip is less satisfactory. It is less satisfactory for rheumatoid arthritis because of the tendency for many joints to be affected. A patient can function reasonably well with two fused wrists but the idea of managing with two fused knees or two fused hips is an appalling prospect.

The best case for fusion of the hip or knee is where only one joint is affected. This is most likely to follow injury, where degeneration of the joint follows disruption of the articulating surfaces. In our present state of knowledge, used carefully, a hip replacement will last some 20 years and a knee replacement approximately 12–15 years. Many serious injuries of the hip and knee occur in young patients — particularly motor cyclists in their late teens. Total joint replacement is not a particularly good idea in these very young patients because such patients lack constraint in any other joint and will be likely to loosen the new joint as a result of excessive activity. How long the new joint will last depends upon the bonding of the implant to the bone, and excessive activity can cause loosening long before the expected 20-year period. Many young motor cyclists will not accept limitation of activity after a total joint replacement and it is preferable in these cases to advise an arthrodesis of the hip or knee as they will have a strong, pain-free joint that will allow them to stand and walk for unlimited periods. In the tall patient, however, travel by car is difficult.

Arthroplasty

A diseased joint may be repaired in four ways:

1. By *excising* the affected joint surfaces and allowing tough scar tissue to form between the bone ends. This is particularly useful for the joints at the base of the toes and results in improved function and pain relief.
2. By *interposing* a layer of another material between the opposing surfaces of a damaged joint. For some years this type of arthroplasty has been applied to the hip by capping the head of the thigh bone with a metal cap (Fig. 5).
3. By *partially replacing* a joint — in the hip and knee where one half of the joint can be replaced (Fig. 6). Thus

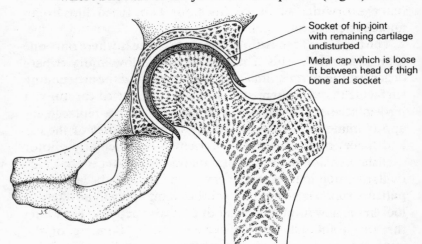

Socket of hip joint with remaining cartilage undisturbed

Metal cap which is loose fit between head of thigh bone and socket

Fig. 5. Interpositional arthroplasty (Smith–Peterson cup).

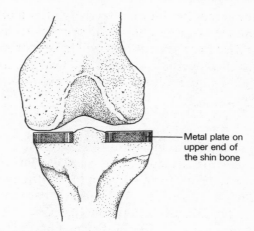

Metal plate on upper end of the shin bone

Fig. 6. Partial knee replacement.

the head of the thigh bone in the hip (see Fig. 7), the lower end of the thigh bone in the knee, or the upper end of the shin bone in the knee (see Fig. 6) may be removed and replaced with a metal insert, moulded to reproduce the original shape of the bone. This idea has been developed over many years producing a number of different designs of insert, usually made of metal.

However, this has the obvious disadvantage in arthritis of only replacing one half of a diseased joint in which both surfaces are damaged, thus leaving a damaged surface articulating with a metal replacement. Nevertheless there are some circumstances where this form of replacement is useful, for example in replacing the head of the thigh bone which has collapsed after a fracture in an elderly person.

4. By *totally replacing* the joint. This is applied to the hip, knee, and finger joints, and is being increasingly applied to the shoulder, ankle, and elbows. In these total joint replacements an attempt is made to produce the low frictional characteristics of the normal human joint by

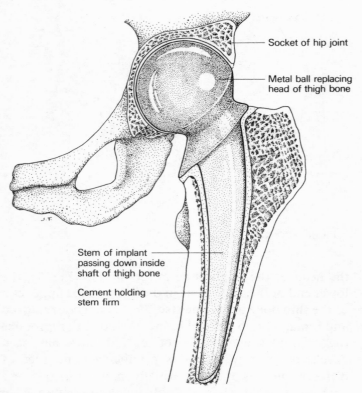

Socket of hip joint

Metal ball replacing head of thigh bone

Stem of implant passing down inside shaft of thigh bone

Cement holding stem firm

Fig. 7. A Thompson prosthesis.

mimicking as closely as possible those surfaces in shape and architecture (Fig. 8).

Nevertheless, the normal human joint produces such a low level of friction between its articulating surfaces that it normally moves freely, smoothly, and without any unpleasant sensation at all. Engineers so far have been unable to produce any with such a low level of friction between the components. Also the very fact that the joint has been opened at operation and part of it replaced means that it can never again be entirely normal. Therefore no-one can pretend that any joint

Operations for degenerative joint disease

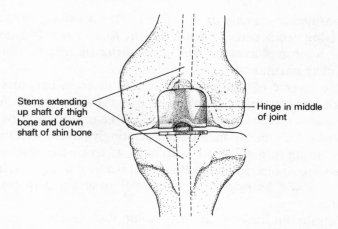

Stems extending up shaft of thigh bone and down shaft of shin bone

Hinge in middle of joint

Fig. 8. Hinge-type knee replacement.

replacement is entirely perfect and certainly at the present time we are not capable of repairing a joint to complete normality.

When we are considering operation on a joint, a total replacement, or another of the other procedures we are mentioning it must be realized that we are expecting a very considerable improvement in the patient's function and not pretending to return the joint to complete normality.

Total joint replacement

This is the most rapidly expanding form of surgery for diseased joints. The surgeon who advises the operation needs to know that the patient is

(a) sufficiently disabled to need the operation;
(b) sufficiently robust to withstand the operation; and
(c) will be sufficiently improved to make use of the replaced joint afterwards.

The ideal case for total joint replacement is the person in their sixties who has good general health and whose disability

Hip replacement: the facts

is confined to one hip or knee joint. This is usually someone suffering from osteoarthritis and in these circumstances a total joint replacement will restore the patient to almost complete normality.

The reverse of this situation occurs where a patient with rheumatoid arthritis in severe degree becomes chair-bound because of advanced disease in one of the major joints of the lower limbs. One hip may be excruciatingly painful and make even sitting in a chair very difficult. If lesser methods have failed a total hip replacement is indicated here solely to relieve pain, in the knowledge that overall function will not be improved.

Certain limitations to total joint replacement must be observed.

1. Preferably the joint being considered for surgical treat-ment should be the cause of the predominant disability, as large numbers of joints cannot be operated upon at any one time.

2. Not every joint is suitable for surgical treatment. The diseased joint may be inaccessible or the presently available methods of replacement contraindicated as they constitute bad engineering.

3. There is a limit to the number of operations any patient can be expected to undergo.

4. In inflammatory polyarthritis (rheumatoid arthritis affecting many joints) an operation can only affect the single joint being subjected to surgery and not cure the entire disease.

    However, often the removal of severe pain from a badly damaged joint can allow a patient to reduce the dosage of steroids and this can result in an improvement in their general health.

5

The technology of joint replacement

The total replacement of the head of the thigh bone and its articulating socket is an accepted practice that has been reached, gradually, as a result of trial and error over many years.

When a joint was disorganized by arthritis and was stiff and painful as a result — the first measures used to rectify the situation were to place a material between the joint surfaces — many materials were used at the beginning of the century varying from skin, to pig's bladder, to gold foil. The factors influencing the result were not fully understood and the results varied enormously — good results being not frequent, but the enthusiasm of the surgeon was to attempt to make every case into a good result. Later in 1937 Smith Peterson of Boston used vitallium, a chrome–cobalt alloy, at the suggestion of his dentist, John Cooke, thus demonstrating the value of airing your problems when seated in the dentist's chair! (Fig. 5).

Total hip replacement was first introduced by Philip Wiles of London in 1938. He used stainless steel components that were fixed by screws and bolts. Further total hip replacements were performed in New York by Haboush in 1953 and Kenneth McKee of Norwich, England in 1951. These implants produced rather poor results because of inadequate fixation, and tended to work loose when walking was resumed.

In 1954 John Charnley observed a patient who had a Judet perspex replacement for the head of the thigh bone for arthritis of the hip. It worked satisfactorily but it gave an audible squeak every time it moved. The patient sought advice because his wife could not bear the sound, it went 'straight through her', so much so that she couldn't even sit at the same table as him, because when he leaned over to pick up the salt his hip emitted a piercing squeak!

This observation led John Charnley to think that the basic fault with the current attempts at joint replacement was deficient lubrication. He consulted the literature on the lubrication of animal joints and found that very little work had been carried out on the subject.

The frictional resistance between the surfaces in a joint depends upon how much of those surfaces touch — the less they touch the more easily the two surfaces slide over each other. The amount of force tending to drive the surfaces together, that is the load applied to the joint, has an effect on how easy it is to move one surface over the other. The constant factor that relates load and frictional resistance is obtained by dividing load into the force of frictional resistance. Thus it is a unitless measure by which the frictional resistance of various bearings can be compared and is independent of the amount of surface area in contact.

Lubricants act to keep the surfaces apart. A well-oiled bearing moves more easily than a dry one. Two mechanisms function at the cartilage surfaces to maintain lubrication. In so-called *boundary lubrication*, molecules of the synovial fluid attach themselves by chemical interaction to the cartilage surfaces. These bound molecules create a boundary layer which when rubbed together offer less resistance to sheer forces than would two dry articular surfaces rubbing against each other. This situation is similar to the wax coating placed on the bottom of skis to make them slippery and run more easily (Fig. 9(a)). In joints the boundary layer is too fragile to withstand high forces, and the lubricant cannot be held in place under the conditions that exist in the joint in repetitive movements such as walking or running.

In most bearings, the lubricant is held in place by the physical force generated by the sliding action of the bearing pushing the lubricant ahead, and this mechanism of *hydrodynamic*

The technology of joint replacement

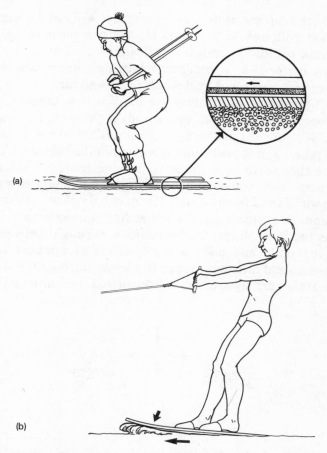

Fig. 9. (a) Boundary lubrication. The wax on the ski and the water on the ice create a boundary layer which when rubbed together offer little resistance. (b) Hydrodynamic lubrication. The water-ski is an example of hydrodynamic lubrication where the ski pushes a wedge of fluid in front of it and motion is maintained as a result of this.

lubrication depends upon the relative motion of the surfaces to maintain a wedge of fluid lubricant. Water-skiing depends upon a wedge of water being pushed in front of the ski — if speed is not sufficient to maintain the relative motion of the ski on the surface of the water the wedge will not develop and the ski will sink (Fig. 9(b)). Hydrodynamic lubrication is unsuited for joints because a lubricating wedge of fluid cannot be maintained in an oscillating bearing, that is one that is moving forwards and backwards as in walking.

In joints, the lubricating mechanism that appears to be present under high loads and speeds is 'weeping lubrication' (Fig. 10). Instead of the fluid being pushed forward into the contact area, it is pushed up from within the substance of the contacting surfaces themselves. As the joint is loaded the lubricant in the zone of potential contact is pressurized and the interstitial fluid from cartilage is squeezed out of the cartilage around the periphery of the impending contact area.

As the joint slides, the 'wept fluid' is caught between the moving parts and adds a low-viscosity component to the synovial fluid already trapped in the area, aiding the separation of the cartilage surfaces. Pressurized fluid or hydrostatic

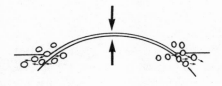

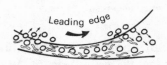

Fig. 10. Weeping lubrication. This occurs where fluid is pushed out of the articulating surfaces on to the contact area. The load is taken on the joint, fluid is squeezed out of the cartilage around the edge of the area of contact.

The technology of joint replacement

lubrication is an effective way of maintaining fluid and position against an external load. In industry, pumps are used to maintain hydrostatic pressure, whereas in joints the articular cartilage under load self-generates pressure which squeezes the fluid in the cartilage out on to the surface.

During a normal cycle of joint motion, one would expect the prevalent lubricating mechanism continually to change from predominantly boundary to predominantly 'weeping' back to predominantly boundary with a combination of both mechanisms active during most of the load and motion cycle.

Charnley went on to measure the coefficient of friction of the human knee joint and obtained an average value of 0.013 which is extremely low, being one-third of that for ice sliding on ice (0.03) and between a tenth and a twentieth of that for a polished steel surface moving over lubricated brass bearings (0.1–0.2). A coefficient of friction of 0.01 means that a load of 100 lb (i.e. a small adult weighing 100 lb) could be made to slide by applying a force of 1 lb.

This remarkably low coefficient of friction of animal joints is helped by the peculiar properties of synovial fluid: it is remarkably tenacious and resistant to rupture.

From those studies, John Charnley wanted to find a material that would behave like normal articular cartilage with its low frictional characteristics, irrespective of what fluid may be on the surface. He ideally wanted a self-lubricating substance.

The most slippery substance known to man at that time was polytetrafluorethylene (p.t.f.e.) or Teflon, which was and is still used to coat non-stick frying pans. The substance had a coefficient of friction of about 0.04 when used against itself or stainless steel. It was found to be exceptionally inert when implanted into the body. The main disadvantage was that it had low physical strength, and had to be used in thick pieces because it behaved like a dense wax, in that deformation took place where thin layers were used.

Charnley used this material in 1958 in the first hip replace-

Hip replacement: the facts

ment, using different materials for the socket and for the head. This was the first time that this had been done in medicine, usually any attempts at fashioning a joint in surgery had employed similar materials for both sides of the joint. I asked him why he had chosen different materials and he replied that sound engineering practice had always dictated different materials, the commonest example being the crankshaft of the automobile where the journals of cast iron articulate with the white-metal bearings in the crank.

The results of those early operations were remarkable for the relief of pain and freedom of movement without any muscle spasm. Charnley, eager and enthusiastic, performed 300 of the operations but kept the procedure under his own personal control, and this was shown to be justified because after 12–18 months the initial early success began to deteriorate. It was found that the plastic shed off into the joint began to cause an irritation of the joint lining to produce a boggy swelling of the joint. This phenomenon could not be predicted because material that had been implanted into experimental animals had failed to produce any local reaction.

These were terrible times for John Charnley.

The early promise of the procedure had been short lived and he shared in the patients' disappointment when their remarkable period of relief of pain began to revert to their pre-operative level. He developed an aversion to the plastic articulation and started work on a sealed silicone hip unit that would have been a purely mechanical solution to the pressing problem of the day — degenerative hip disease. At this time, Lady Luck intervened. A salesman came into the laboratory with a sample of a new material and showed it to the technician. Whereas the material previously used was low-density polyethylene (p.t.f.e.) this new material was produced as a result of more tightly compacting, or polymerizing the plastic, and it was called high density polyethylene (h.d.p.). The technician presented this new material to Charnley — who, very mindful of the Teflon failure, told him with some Anglo-

30

The technology of joint replacement

Saxon endorsements, to throw it away! The technician, Harry Craven, returned to the laboratory rather crestfallen, and looked at the wear-testing machine standing idle and gathering dust. He put the sample of h.d.p. on to the machine and left it running. At the end of three weeks he found that there was less wear than there had been after one day with p.t.f.e. He showed the results to Charnley, who instructed him to make up some cups for further experimentation.

The first cups of the new material were implanted in November 1962 and there have been 20 000 operations performed since then at Wrightington alone, with upwards of 2 000 000 performed throughout the world successfully (Fig. 11).

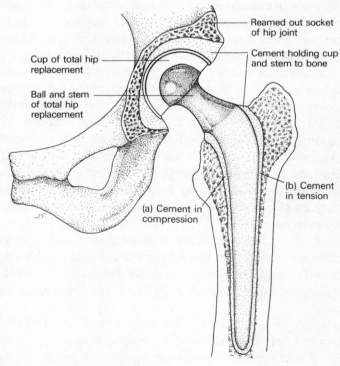

Fig. 11.   Total hip replacement.

Hip replacement: the facts

What of those patients who had had the Teflon operation? Charnley revised 95 per cent of those operations himself. One of the early residents told me that it was like observing a monk pouring ashes over his own head each time he revised a case, but it was a measure of the relief of pain afforded by the first procedure that such a high proportion of the patients were willing to submit themselves to a second operation.

We talk of the Teflon failure and much comment is made these days about experimentation in medicine — guinea-pigs — the anti-vivisectionists are even objecting to guinea-pigs being used as guinea-pigs. But was the Teflon experience a failure? In later life John Charnley looked at that time more philosophically. He said that the whole technology of the procedure was worked out in the Teflon era: the clean air, cement technique, operative instruments, and design of implant refined. All of this work was ready when the right material came along. The vast majority of the patients had a revision of their Teflon cups and were restored to worthwhile function. These patients knew that they were sharing a new surgical technology and the possibility of failure was explained to them beforehand. The poor results from the currently practised hip operations of the day made them willing to take a measured risk, knowing that they could not be worse after the operation and had the possibility of being very much improved. They shared the disappointment of John Charnley at the setback, but they had enough faith in him to allow him to perform a second operation.

Those 300 pioneer patients enabled a new technology to become established that has now given relief to 10 000 times that number and ushered in the era of modern joint replacement surgery, where fear of crippling joint disease has been removed.

Haboush in 1952 had used acrylic cement for fitting the implant but only in small amounts, considering it an adhesive. It was Charnley who developed the use of acrylic cement recognizing that it had to be used in large amounts. Previous

The technology of joint replacement

cement techniques used it as a glue or adhesive because it was used in small amounts as an adjuvant to a tight mechanical fit of the implant in the bone. Charnley felt this was wrong because the tight mechanical fit would cause the bone to absorb the cement and then leave the implant unsupported by an inadequate amount of cement. He taught the radical step of making the implant a loose fit in the bone at the time of surgery so as to have cement interposed on all surfaces. Acrylic cement as he used it was a 'grout' and not an adhesive. A grout is a material that bonds surfaces together by producing mechanical interference, whereas an adhesive reacts chemically with the surface to produce its effect. Using acrylic cement to fix the stems of prostheses in the thigh bone he was able to demonstrate that it improved the bond by over 200 times compared to conventional fixation without cement. Cement fixation can be achieved successfully in bone that is soft and porous because the load of the weight of the body is distributed over such a large area.

The metal part of the total hip replacement consisting of the ball which articulates with the artificial socket, and the stem which passes down the inside of the shaft of the thigh bone, has many demands on its function. The bone that it replaces is tubular consisting of an outer surface of hard cortical bone which gives way on the inside to a meshwork of soft bone called cancellous bone. The metal prosthesis is of course solid and does not have the variable structure of the bone that it replaces. It has not been possible so far to mimic the anatomical structure of the head of the thigh bone solely because it is not possible at this stage of engineering development to create a joint with such low frictional characteristics as the normal human joint.

The early stems were quite slender affairs and breakage did occur in some cases. It was as a result of this breakage that the forces that were imparted to the joints of the body began to be studied. It was not realized at first that up to three times body weight could be transmitted through the hip joint, and the early implants were not able to withstand these very large forces. Ideally the metal replacing the head and neck of the thigh bone would have the same strength as the bone and also the same elasticity. Bone is a living structure and does move, that is flex, during activity even though the amounts of movement are very small. If a metal is too flexible it will eventually be subjected to fatigue failure and break. If a metal is too stiff, its bonding within the bone will become weak and it will be subject to loosening. It is in an attempt to have a metal that is sufficiently flexible to move with the bone but sufficiently rigid to withstand high stress that a compromise has had to be reached. If we had an extremely heavy and stiff stem in the thigh bone, repeated use in walking would bring about loosening. If a metal was very flexible it would then be subjected to bending and breakage. Improvements in the design of the stem in the thigh bone, taking into account the stress which will be expended on it, are limited by the internal diameter of the shaft of the thigh bone. The stems that are at present in use, however, are up to nine times as strong as the original rather flimsy stems used in 1958. This increase in strength came about as a result of changes in shape and the advances in metallurgy. These improvements have been the result of research and development by the implant industry so that there is an increased life expectancy from the joint implant.

As a result of the experience of wear in Teflon it was felt that the total hip replacement would last as long as it took for the plastic of the socket to become worn down. High density polyethylene has shown itself to be extremely resistant to wear, and in addition the minute particles formed as a result of wear are not irritant to the surrounding tissues, so that there is no joint reaction after long use, now in many cases up to 20 years.

Limitation of the implant is imposed by the bonding of the implant to the bone both on the stem side and on the socket side. The socket and stem will work loose before they will wear out. Improved bonding of the implants is possible with high pressure injection of the cement into the bone bed. The long-term stability of the total joint replacement is dependent upon using acrylic cement in large quantities to act as a grout, as originally advised by John Charnley.

6

The prevention of infection: ultra-clean air

Total joint replacement involves the insertion of a relatively large implant into the body which is enclosed in the normal body tissues. The area of the implant, usually held in place by bone cement, constitutes an artificial environment which is known to encourage the growth of bacteria. The operation can be a long procedure involving three or four people at the operating site with a similar number outside the immediate operating site in the support team.

Infection has always been a hazard of all types of surgery, but whereas after an abdominal operation during which no foreign material is inserted, a mild infection can resolve as a result of natural resistance, this natural protection is not sufficient after implant surgery, be it vascular or orthopaedic.

In the early days of implant surgery the infection rate was around 10 per cent. Stringent measures had always been taken to sterilize the instruments in high pressure ovens (autoclaves) and the skin was similarly prepared by careful shaving of hair and antiseptic applications to rid the operating site of infecting organisms. It was sterilization of the air that came into contact with both patient and instruments that occupied John Charnley's mind in 1958.

The zone in which the surgical team work and which must also accommodate the instruments is four metres square. In a conventional operating theatre with an air conditioning system, clean air enters at the ceiling and is directed down on to the operating site (Fig. 12a). Warm objects create up-currents, hot objects create rapid up-currents. These always start from the floor which, even in the operating theatre, is bacterially dirty. During average activity a person emits

36

The prevention of infection: ultra-clean air

approximately 10 000 bacteria-carrying particles per minute and on them ride all the bacteria which are to be found on the body. The footwear of the operating theatre personnel scuff the floor, pushing contaminants into the air. These are induced by convection to rise upwards and combine with the bacteria carrying particles being emitted by the operating team, and which are in turn transported on the convection up-currents from their own warm bodies.

Movement of hands, arms, and bodies create considerable turbulence so that they deflect these contaminated air currents in all directions, infecting the wound directly, and also, indirectly, by contaminating the gloves and instruments which go into the wound (Fig. 12(c)).

Heat generated by the operating lamp will induce these con-taminated up-currents to accelerate to a speed between 10 and 15 metres per minute, depending on the type of lamp used and whether it has its own integral heat exhaust system to cool it.

At this relatively high speed the contaminants reach the ceiling where they are carried along the flow of clean air enter-ing the operating room from the conventional air conditioning

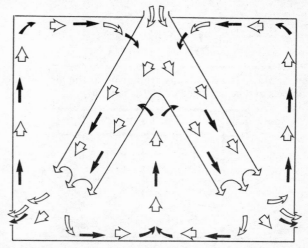

Fig. 12(a) Air flow in conventional operating theatre with ceiling diffuser.

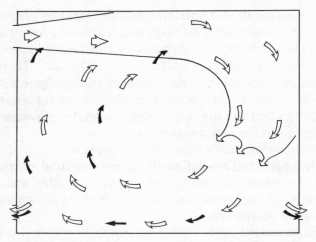

(b) A side-wall diffuser (light arrows indicate clean air and dark arrows bacterially contaminated air from the floor).

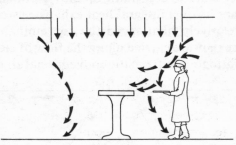

(c) Laminar flow. If side-screens are not used, the air will flow round moving objects and be deflected on to the patient.

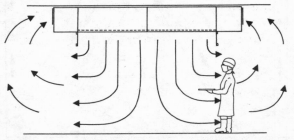

(d) Exponential flow. Even when side-screens are not used in the 'tent' air is not deflected on to the patient.

Fig. 12.

diffusers, which unfortunately recycles them downwards again on to the open operating wound. The results with clean air coming in from one of the side walls is just as bad (Fig. 12(b)).

Charnley realized that it was necessary to produce a circulation of air in the theatre that combated the upward rising convection current and did not draw bacteria from the floor and spread it across the wound. It was also necessary to avoid turbulence of the air.

A fruitful collaboration began between John Charnley and Hugh Howarth, an air engineer. Howarth was a third-generation air engineer whose family firm had specialized in making air conditioning systems for large textile mills which were designed to avoid dust in the atmosphere and air purification systems for the brewing industry which were designed to prevent stray yeasts getting into the beer. The problem of clean air in an area of four square metres presented little technical difficulty. They devised an enclosure within the standard operating theatre which produced a sterile environment for the lower two-thirds of the patient, and there was room inside the enclosure for only those people (three or four) immediately concerned with the operation. Even the anaesthetist was kept outside in order to reduce to a minimum the unsterile dust particles generated over the open wound.

The clean air was to enter the enclosure through a porous ceiling that could itself be sterilized along with the filtration system. This small enclosure within the larger operating theatre was often referred to as 'the tent' (Fig. 12(d)).

Respirators were to be worn inside the enclosure so that the surgeon's expired air could be evacuated through exhaust tubes to right outside the enclosure (Fig. 13(b)). A surgeon working inside such an enclosure would no longer have instruments put into his hand as in a conventional theatre. The standard practice in surgery is for all of the instruments to be laid out on a trolley and to be used as necessary. This established practice could not be allowed in the small

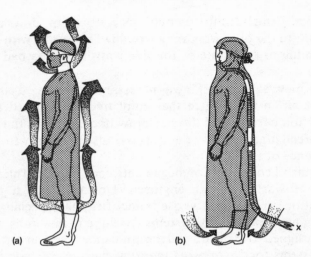

Fig. 13. (a) A conventional operating suit. Arrows indicate convection currents carrying organisms. (b) Charnley–Howarth all-enveloping operating gown with body exhaust. All convection currents from the surgeon are exhausted through the tube at x.

enclosure and John Charnley devised the tray system. He divided the operation up into seven natural stages and all instruments necessary were placed on separate trays so that when stage one was over the first tray was passed out and was replaced by a new tray with all the instruments for stage two. This standardization of technique has enabled an excellent theatre discipline to evolve so that over 30 hips can be operated upon in a normal working week. The surgeons and assistants inside the enclosure wear all-enclosing gowns and helmets with clear plastic visors — so that their exhalations and secretions are aspirated to the outside of the enclosure (Fig. 13(b)).

The gowns are made of fine Sudanese cotton with a very small weave called Ventyl. In any operation the surgeon's gown can become moist through perspiration on the inside or blood and fluid on the outside. In standard material this leads to high permeability in the same way that wind is always felt more keenly if one is wearing a shirt that has been wet for any

The prevention of infection: ultra-clean air

reason. High permeability would normally allow the passage of organisms, but the Ventyl material has a valuable property: when it becomes moist the fine fibres swell so that the permeability remains low and this potential source of infection is lost.

The small enclosure is thus continuously swept by air moving in a downwards direction and this uniform, unidirectional flow of air is called laminar flow. If an attempt was made to produce laminar flow in the whole theatre as opposed to the small enclosure, a huge pump and mechanical plant would be necessary with the consequent usage of a large amount of energy. In a further refinement of laminar flow Hugh Howarth varied the speed of the air flow within the enclosure so that it was most rapid over the patient and gradually reduced towards the edges. The idea for this last refinement came to him on holiday. He had not taken a holiday for two years and was spending a few days in Barbados. As was his custom he lay beneath a palm tree on the beach with his usual drawing pad whilst his wife lay in the sun alongside him. The idea came to him as he visualized the air pattern that emitted from the trumpet in the dance band of the night before. He was unable to get into his holiday and thoroughly relax until he had sent off telexes to his company offices in Bolton, England, to draw up a patent specification to be ready on his arrival home. In this way it was possible to use the clean-air enclosure without sides, as the air could only go in one direction, without the danger of unsterile air entering from outside.

The total inability of a conventional air-conditioning system to control air behaviour patterns and so prevent the dissemination of airborne contamination was confirmed by a study which measured the number of bacteria-carrying particles per cubic centimetre at the wound site with various air systems. It produced the data shown in Table 1.

Hip replacement: the facts

Table 1

Operating theatre air system and type of clothing	Conditions at the site of the operation	
	Air flow pattern speed	Bacteria-carrying particles per metre
Conventionally air conditioned 8–10 persons — conventional gowns and masks	Not under control, turbulent	400–500
Horizontal air flow, 8–10 persons wearing conventional gowns and masks	Laminar, 20 metres per minute	34
Downwards air flow 8–10 persons wearing conventional gowns and masks	Laminar, 20 metres per minute	8
Downwards air flow with Charnley Howarth Total Body Exhaust System	Laminar, 20 metres per minute	0.63

This figure of 0.63 bacteria-carrying particles measured at the site of the incision represents a reduction of over 650 times when compared with a conventional well air-conditioned operating theatre. There can be no doubt that surgeons and theatre nursing staff are conservative in inclination in that they not only know what they like, but they also like what they know. The total body exhaust system and clean air enclosure can look strange and forbidding to the uninitiated but it is certainly comfortable and refreshing to work in. There was indifference bordering at times on hostility to the clean air enclosure technique. Sometimes discussions could get quite heated. Some surgeons state that an ordinary theatre is quite satisfactory and prophylactic antibiotics are all that is necessary. I have compared this to the situation where you know that a particular restaurant has dirty kitchens and when you dine you take the precaution of sprinkling antiseptic on the salad.

The difficulty lay in statistically proving that the clean air enclosure was worthwhile. As a result of the continuous refinements in technique and theatre practice the infection rate at Wrightington has gradually fallen to less than 0.5 per cent.

The prevention of infection: ultra-clean air

Table 2

Wrightington hospital's record of the reduction of infection

System	Year	Colonies/plate/hr	Total No. of Operations	Infections (%)
Conventional theatre with exhaust ventilation	1959–1961	80–90	190	7.0
First prototype enclosure Electro-static filter	1962	25	108	3.7
Second prototype Howarth donated system	1963–1965	1.8	1079	2.2
Howarth permanent Enclosure Mk.1	1966–1968	0 (limit of accuracy)	1929	1.5
Howarth Permanent Enclosures Mk 1 and Mk 2 and	1969–1970 1971–1972	0 0	2125 over 2000	0.5 0.3
Howarth Demount-able System	1973–1976	0	over 4000	0.3
Running total	1969–1981		over 17 000	0.3 to 0.5

The importance and validity of the statistics shown in Table 2 will be appreciated more fully when it is realized that:

1. *No antibiotics* were given to the patient before the operation.
2. All patients maintain contact with the hospital and are observed for a minimum period of *three years* after the operation.

In order to have valid statistical evidence for the benefit of clean air zones, a large number of patients need to be operated upon and patients randomly assigned to be operated on in conventional theatres or clean air enclosures.

In 1974 the Hospital Inspection Committee of the Medical Research Council of Great Britain recommended that a controlled investigation be carried out. It was considered that between 7000 and 8000 operations would have to be followed in order to reach an acceptable probability (90 per cent) of detecting with reasonable certainty (at the 95 per cent confidence level) a reduction in the infection risk from 2 per cent to 1 per cent for either or both of the two options (a) 'ultra clean' air alone or (b) 'ultra clean' air together with the wearing of whole body exhaust suits. The latter as well as reducing the level of airborne bacterial contamination, reduces the chance of direct transfer of microorganisms into the wound from the surgeon's skin.

Conclusive evidence has now been reported from this study on over 8000 operations carried out between 1974 and 1979 — the incidence of joint infection was approximately half for those operations performed in an ultra-clean air system compared with that observed where a conventionally ventilated theatre was used. The wearing of the whole body exhaust suits in the ultra-clean air environment was associated with an even greater reduction, to less than one quarter.

The present design of Charnley–Howarth enclosure no longer looks like a tent, but there can be no doubt about the benefit it confers on total joint replacement.

7

How to prepare for the operation

If symptoms are intermittent you should try to remain as active as possible to keep the muscles in good tone. If an operation has been advised your surgeon will need to ensure that your general health is sufficiently good to enable you to withstand the operation and that you are robust enough to be able to benefit from it afterwards. At the time of surgery, you need to be in good physical shape because of the hard work needed afterwards in walking with crutches or a stick.

Your weight must be satisfactory — if you are overweight it will be difficult to manage walking with either crutches or sticks afterwards. A fat abdomen makes rising from a chair difficult. A robust, healthy patient once rebuked me for not telling him to lose weight before the operation as he felt sorry for the nurses who had to lift him afterwards! To reduce weight and prepare for the operation a varied diet containing plenty of green vegetables and fresh fruit with first-class protein is advisable. Your physician will check that you are not anaemic. Moderation would dictate a gradual reduction of weight over many months to avoid the loss of strength and vigour that can arise from rapid loss of weight.

Your lungs need to be clear for the anaesthetic agent. Generally anaesthetists do not like heavy smokers, particularly cigarette smokers, as this makes the lungs sensitive to anaesthetic agents and can lead to bronchial spasm and breathlessness. You should attempt to reduce cigarette smoking — or preferably stop smoking altogether! Blood pressure needs to be within normal limits so as not to put too much pressure on the heart during the operation — this will be checked by your anaesthetist before the operation. It is recognized that a gradual increase in blood pressure occurs with age, and even when blood pressure is abnormally high, effective treatment by your physician enables surgery to be performed safely.

Active infection is a contraindication to surgery, for example teeth abscesses can cause the bacteria to circulate in the bloodstream, and settle on the joint implant. Urinary tract infection, particularly if necessitating a catheter post-operatively, can be associated with infection of the implant and your surgeon will be anxious to clean up any urinary tract infections or bladder obstruction before surgery.

Treatment of any site of infection will depend upon the type of organism that is causing the infection and your physician will prescribe the appropriate antibiotics for the relevant period.

It is generally advisable to allow at least three to four weeks to elapse after active antibiotic treatment to ensure everything has settled down before proceeding with your joint replacement. Remember that with hip replacement the life of your new joint should be 20 years and with knee replacement probably up to 12 years (in our present state of knowledge). So it is unwise to want to rush things for a matter of a few weeks when a long period of benefit is expected.

General medical conditions such as diabetes, kidney failure, and heart failure, do not constitute a contraindication to total joint replacement as long as the appropriate precautions are taken, thanks to modern highly skilled anaesthetic techniques, with monitoring of vital bodily functions, such as heart rate and pattern of contraction, blood gases, and central venous pressure.

Drug treatment of rheumatoid arthritis and other diseases with an allergic basis often involves the prescription of steroids. It is important that the anaesthetist is given details of steroid treatment, even if treatment has ceased for many years, as there may well be a need for extra steroids during the operation and recovery period.

How to prepare for the operation

The younger female patients may be taking oral contraceptive pills — these will need to be stopped for four weeks prior to surgery, and the risks of conception avoided so as to prevent the complications of thrombo-embolism (blood clots) associated with the pill and operations.

EXERCISE BEFORE THE HIP OPERATION

Long periods of disuse are as bad as over exertion for a joint affected by osteoarthritis. Walk little and often and don't be too proud to use a walking stick. You will not only be helping to exercise the muscles of the joint involved, but also keeping the heart in good tone. Spells of cold, damp weather make the joint capsule stiff so be prepared to keep your home warm and wear extra clothing.

Weight-bearing exercise such as walking can cause pain, but how much pain will vary from person to person. It is not advisable to continue activity that is causing pain *within the joint*. Useful methods of exercise that are non-weight-bearing are swimming and cycling. It is unusual for someone to take sufficient exercise by swimming — three to four lengths of a 50 metre pool is not enough to sufficiently stress the hip muscles, because the swimmer usually experiences breathlessness before this. There will of course be people who are expert swimmers who are able to gain useful exercise in this way.

Many more people will be able to take useful exercise by riding a bicycle — which is usually more available and less time consuming. The stationary exercise bicycle is very convenient, but is less interesting than getting around on an ordinary bicycle. Individual circumstances will vary. For some, because of traffic conditions, poor hearing or eyesight, or living in an unsuitable area, the stationary cycle is best. In any case the opportunity to indulge in strenuous exercise that does not result in pain within the joint is a great relief. By way of example, a 28-year-old mother of two came to see me suffering with degenerative arthritis of the hip, secondary to congenital dislocation of the hip as an infant. She was finding it increasingly difficult to run her household, take her children to and from school, and do her shopping. In addition, she had an emotional problem in that towards the end of the day she felt so tired and her hip ached so much that she needed large doses of anti-inflammatory analgesics to enable her to sleep so that she could not contemplate sexual relations, and as a result tension was developing between her and her husband. The use of a bicycle strengthened the hip muscles and completely changed her life, so that she could cope with her chores, the hip ceased to drag her down, and she became a completely changed person, obviously coping with all reasonable activities, being able to dispense altogether with pain killers.

In the later stage of hip disease, the joint loses its articular cartilage as it becomes worn and the leg becomes shorter as a result of loss of true length. The joint loses movement and the capsule becomes thickened and stiff. The leg becomes drawn across the midline (adducted), and drawn forwards (flexed) and this causes a further shortening as a result of loss of apparent length. You cannot stand with your foot stuck up in the air, so it is brought to the ground by bending the knee and hitching the buttocks. The final deformity is the whole leg turning outward (external rotation) evidenced by the foot turning outwards.

The stride length will be reduced as well as the ability to separate the ankles, this latter leading to a reduction in ability to regain balance after stumbling — you cannot put your foot out to save yourself as well as before — the whole causing a loss of confidence and desire to walk outside the home.

The following exercises are advocated:

Capsular stretching exercise to combat flexion deformity (Fig. 14)

1. Place two dining chairs back to back, but the width of the body apart.

How to prepare for the operation

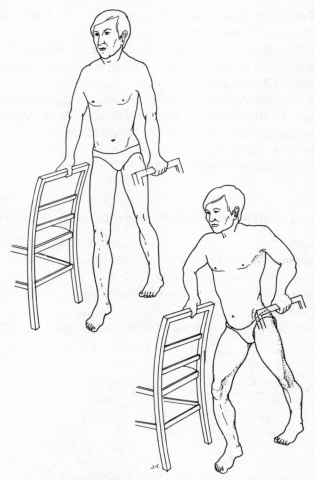

Fig. 14. Capsular stretching exercise to combat flexion deformity.

2. Place one hand and forearm on the back of each chair to take some body weight.
3. Place the affected leg behind you, with the leg and knee held straight and the heel on the ground with the foot pointing forwards.

4. The front foot now will be between the backs of the chairs at about midway.
5. Bending the front knee and arching the back will cause weight to be swung on to the affected hip tending to stretch it straight.
6. As you become accustomed to the exercise more weight can be brought on to the affected limb by taking gradually less weight on the forearms.
7. Repeat 30 times each session.
8. Do at least six sessions daily.

Stretching exercise to increase ankle separation (Fig. 15)

1. Stand with your ankles as far apart as possible. Keep the knees straight and the toes pointing forwards.
2. Place your hands on your hips.
3. Bend the non- (or less) affected knee forwards and outwards.
4. Swing your body weight over to this side by pressing

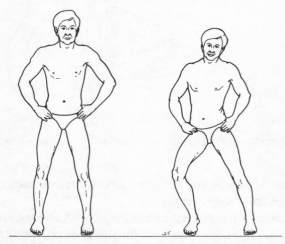

Fig. 15. Stretching exercise of left hip to increase ankle separation.

your hand into the bad hip and pushing downwards and towards the non-affected side.

5. Straighten up to position in (1).
6. Repeat this exercise up to 30 times each session, gradually increasing the intensity.

Correction of external rotation deformity to keep foot straight

If both of the preceding exercises have been performed keeping the foot pointing forwards as much as possible, then improvement in this deformity will occur without any specific measures.

Of course, gradual deterioration of the joint occurs in the large majority of patients with arthritis of the hip, even when these exercises are done, but such exercises have many purposes. They can provide a holding action in what had previously been a deteriorating condition and help to make the pain more tolerable. They can improve matters when surgery has to be delayed while some other medical condition is cleared up. The exercises improve the condition of the muscles and capsule and are of benefit as a starting-point in rehabilitation after joint replacement.

In some cases they may so improve symptoms that operation can be postponed indefinitely. Who wants to have an operation if it can be avoided? A good surgeon knows when not to operate!

In many cases, these exercises will be performed where patients are taking pain-relieving pills — 'pain killers' — analgesics. One group of drugs, the anti-inflammatory analgesics, are very useful in suppressing the pain and aching in the early stages of the degenerative joint condition. Indeed, in many patients the hip or knee joint degeneration is part of a generalized joint condition and the anti-inflammatory analgesics are an invaluable agent in making life bearable. They are a good servant and a poor master, and never cure the degenerative condition. They should not be taken in order to facilitate exercise activity as they will have the effect of masking the pain that would normally occur in the joint and lead the patient to break off the activity. If this natural protection is masked by pain killers, there is a tendency to accelerate the wearing down of the joint surface. In this situation, the pills can have the effect of causing accelerated wear and tear. Anti-inflammatory analgesics are intended to make bearable reasonable daily living activities such as walking, going up and down stairs, and getting in and out of chairs and cars. They are not to be taken to allow someone to take up jogging!

Patients are often obliged to carry out these exercises by themselves.

Progress in combating flexion deformity is measured by increased stride length, and in combating adduction deformity by ankle separation; progress in improving external rotation is self-evident.

Exercises to strengthen the knee (Fig. 16)

The knee is a superficial joint, and not covered with heavy muscles as the the hip is. Its mobility is permitted by virtue of its shape, as it consists of two large 'flat' balls on the lower end of the thigh bone, and two shallow dished sockets on the upper end of the shin bone. Its mobility and exposed position make it liable to injury and wear and tear of the bone ends and the ligaments. Unlike the hip joint, it does benefit from the application of external supports, which can be made from anything from simple elasticated tubing to rigid plastic splints.

Supports of the knee do give comfort in the eary stages of degeneration, but they should never take the place of that support to the knee which comes from strong muscle activity; loss of muscle activity, as with the hip, does arise from loss of leverage in the joint, but this can to a large extent be counteracted by carrying out exercises to strengthen the quadriceps muscle — straight leg raising (Fig. 16).

52

How to prepare for the operation

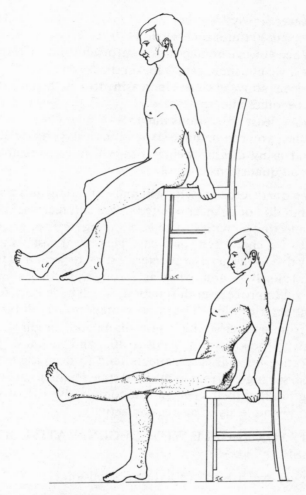

Fig. 16. Straight leg raising exercise.

1. Sit with your bottom at the edge of a chair to allow your affected leg to be as straight as possible. Put your heel on the floor.
2. Lift your foot until your leg is horizontal.
3. Hold for two seconds.

4. Lower slowly.
5. Repeat 30 times each session.
6. When you can manage this comfortably put a weight bag or a weight shoe, say, 2 lb, on the foot.
7. Repeat above exercises increasing to 4 lb then 6 lb when it becomes manageable.
8. Do at least six sessions daily.
9. When you can manage six sessions a day, doing 30 lifts and using a 6 lb* weight you will have re-established good quadriceps control.

Strong quadriceps muscles will make standing and walking easier, but do not be disappointed if you still feel weakness in the 'connecting activities' such as climbing stairs or getting in and out of a chair, bed, or a car. This 'weakness' is unfortunately due to the persistent deterioration or wear and tear in the joint itself — and whereas strong quadriceps muscle power will improve overall function, it will have no effect on the joint deterioration. The improvement in overall function comes from greater strength in walking and standing and in this activity the knee only bends to 40°, and we know that in degenerative knee disease patients tend to decrease even on this modest range, so that in the final stages patients are in fact walking holding their knee almost completely stiff, which is very tiring and leads to decreasing activity.

DON'TS FOR PEOPLE WITH DEGENERATIVE JOINT DISEASE

Don't over exercise or strain the affected joint.

Don't stand or walk for long periods if the hip or knee is painful.

---

*6 lb weight is the average for most people. Clearly people with severe disability and serious wasting of the muscles will not get up to this level, as well as those persons with less severe disability who have small limbs. On the contrary, many males with large quadriceps muscles will get up to 10–12 lb before they restore reasonable strength to their quadriceps muscles.

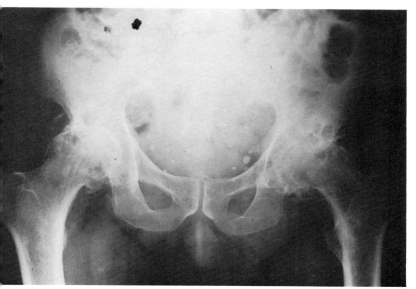

Plate 1(a) Degenerative arthritis of the hip in a 60-year-old man. Severe degenerative change in both hips, the right worse than the left. The patient had been aware of increasing disability for five years, but was only seriously troubled for six months, after which he saw his doctor.

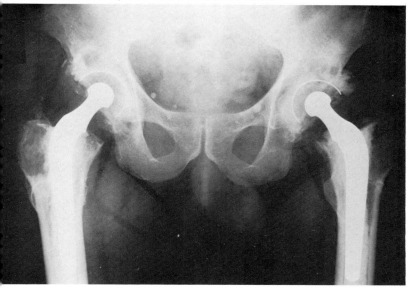

(b) The same patient two years after both hips had been replaced. Excellent function maintained.

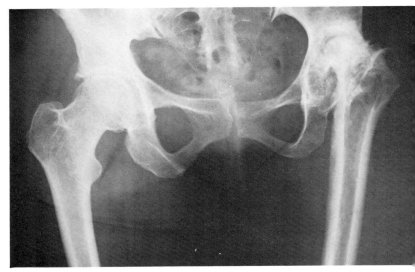

Plate 2(a)   Secondary degenerative arthritis of the left hip following septic arthritis as a child. Note the severe shortening of the left leg.

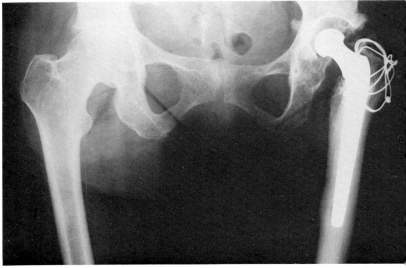

(b)   Left total hip reconstruction produced great relief of pain and markedly increased function, but the patient still needs to wear a raise on her shoe. The operation in this case could not equalize leg length.

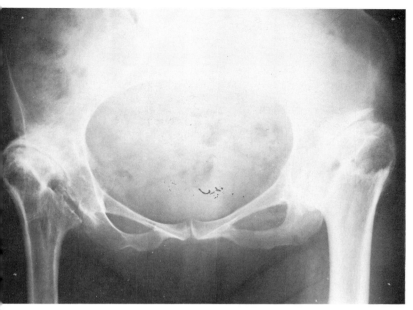

Plate 3(a)   Severe degenerative arthritis of hips secondary to congenital dislocation.

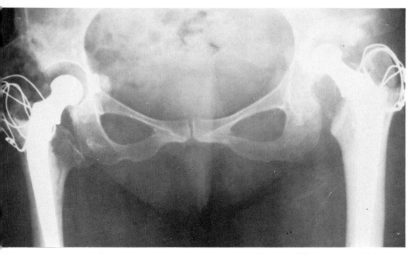

(b)   Bilateral hip replacement greatly increases walking ability and abolishes pain, but these hips do not flex up very high, only 60°. Overall movement is, I think, half of what could be gained in a 'normal' osteoarthritic hip, but overall function very much improved.

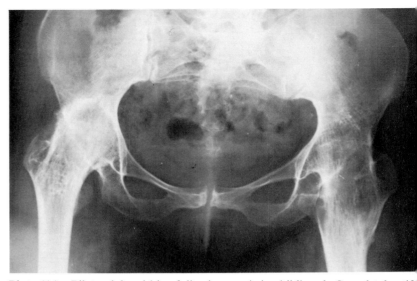

Plate 4(a)   Bilateral fused hips following sepsis in childhood. Completely stiff hipped gait. Great difficulty in manoeuvering chairs, stairs, toilet, etc.

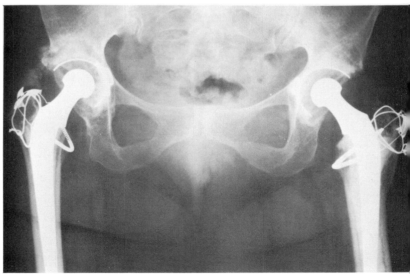

(b)   Following bilateral hip replacement overall function greatly improved, but movement still limited and leg length not equal.

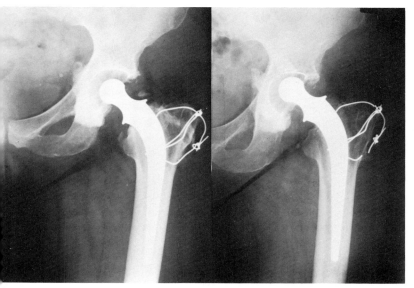

late 5   Left hip replacement carried out in 1964 (*left*) and same patient
8 years later (*right*). Note the wearing out of the cup on the left side. No
ymptoms from this but it is unlikely that the acetabular cups will last more
an 20-25 years.

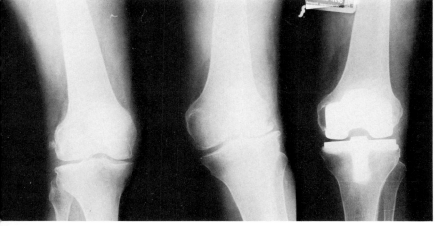

late 6   Severe degenerative arthritis of the knee producing knock-knee
eformity. The third photograph shows alignment of knee restored and pain
elieved by total knee replacement.

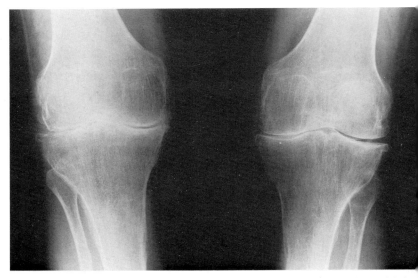

Plate 7(a)   Degenerative arthritis of both knees, producing severe loss of joint space without gross deformity.

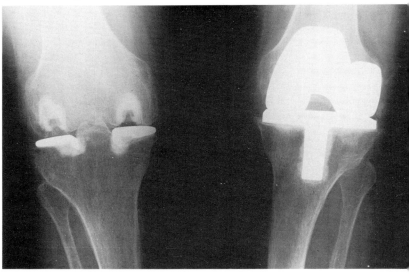

(b)   On the left side, a resurfacing operation has produced reasonable relief of pain, but not a great deal of movement. On the right side a modern resurfacing operation has produced excellent relief of pain and a good range of movement. These two operations represent the progress in total knee replacement over the last 10 years.

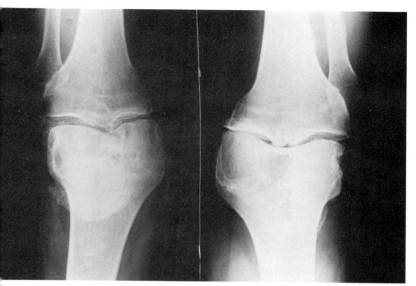

Plate 8   Degenerative arthritis of the knees, the left is worse than the right.

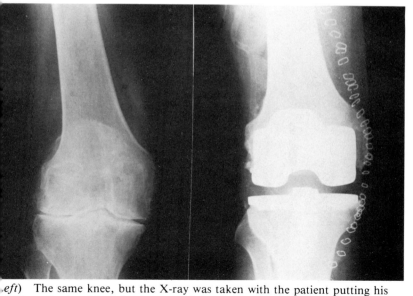

(Left)   The same knee, but the X-ray was taken with the patient putting his weight on the leg. Note the decreased joint space.

(Right)   The same knee after total knee replacement. Alignment is restored. Note temporary clips used to close skin.

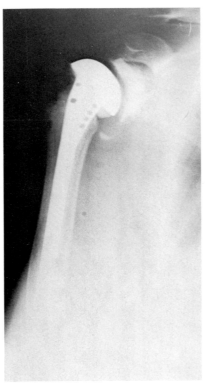

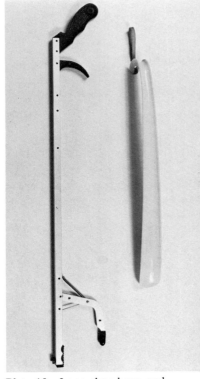

Plate 9   Total shoulder replacement. See Fig. 28. Very satisfactory relief of pain but regaining full range of movement can take many months and intensive physiotherapy is necessary.

Plate 10   Long shoe horn and helping hand device which are a great help in avoiding over-bending the hip in the early stages of recovery.

How to prepare for the operation

Don't be afraid of simple movements to prevent stiffness.

Don't lie or sit for too long in one position.

Don't be too worried by X-ray reports. We treat patients and not X-rays.

Don't listen to advice on diet or wonderful patent medicines and 'cures' — we have no evidence that they work.

8

Total hip replacement: the hospital stay

The following remarks refer to a routine admission for total hip replacement as carried out at Wrightington hospital, which performs the largest number of total joint replacements in the United Kingdom. Practices vary from hospital to hospital and their inclusion or exclusion in this description is not meant to imply criticism. In a similar way we may appear to pay scant respect to some aspects of care which other centres feel are of great importance. Our practice is based on the experience gained in the performance of more than 20 000 total hip replacements from 1958 onwards.

As mentioned earlier, on admission to hospital the patient needs to be in good general health. All patients like to look their best when going into hospital as it can be an unnerving experience, but bear in mind that the purpose of the exercise is to get rid of the pain and to enable a return to useful activity. Do not have an expensive hair-do before going into hospital, since you will be asked to have a shower and wash your whole body, including your hair, with a powerful antiseptic detergent to start the sterilization of the skin before operation.

The general physical examination by the resident doctor will ensure that there are no abnormalities in your central nervous system, chest and heart, abdomen, and genito-urinary system. Blood samples will be taken to establish the normality of these systems in addition to enabling a cross match for blood to be transfused if necessary during surgery. Routine questioning will establish whether you have any allergies to any of the drugs, anaesthetic agents, or lotions that may be used during your hospital stay. Patch testing will be carried out to see if any allergy exists to the antiseptic lotions that will be used for the skin sterilization. You will have a further check by the anaesthetist to ensure that your general condition is acceptable for major surgery.

The day before your operation further skin preparation consists of shaving off the pubic hair and any other hair on the abdomen up to the rib cage as far as the midline, and the whole leg and foot to be operated upon. After shaving it is usual to wear a shift type of gown with side fastenings.

The skin is now sterilized using a compatible antiseptic in a spirit base. You will have two spirit preparations before going to theatre and two more after you are under the anaesthetic. The skin must be free of infection or ulcers.

You will have no further food after midnight on the eve of the operation, and small amounts of fluid by mouth on the day depending upon the time of the operation and the anaesthetist in charge.

Premedication before the operation is usually given in the hour before surgery to enable you to relax and to facilitate the anaesthetic.

You will be given an injection to put you to sleep when you arrive in the anaesthetic room, which is the ante-room to the operating threatre, and you will wake up after a successful operation. You may, however, be interested to know what has been going on while you were asleep.

As mentioned above, a further skin preparation of the whole operation site and lower limb takes place in the anaesthetic room and after transfer to the clean air enclosure the final skin preparation is followed by towelling up with operation drapes to leave only the operation site exposed.

After the skin incision on the side of the thigh the hip joint is exposed by splitting the muscles to bring about dislocation of the head of the thigh bone from the socket. The worn out head is now removed, this also gives easier access to the hip socket.

Special tools are now used to ream out a suitable cavity to accommodate the acetabular cup. This cup clearly needs to vary in size between different patients and the most suitable size is chosen from a study of the X-rays and trial sizes in the actual bony socket cavity. When the bone cavity has been prepared, acrylic cement is introduced into it and pressure is applied to obtain an intimate bond of the cement to the bone of the socket. The cup is then pressed into the cement so that there is no movement between the cup, the acrylic cement, and the hip socket. There is no adhesive property in the cement. It is a grout and holds secure by pushing into the fine honeycomb meshwork of the bone in the hip socket.

Once the cup has been secured, the ball is now put in place after suitable preparation of the shaft of the thigh bone. The ball is contained on the end of a stem and the stem fits down the central cavity of the thigh bone. Once again trial stems are used to see which one fits inside the thigh bone most accurately. The size of the stem varies and the length of the neck of the stem also varies, so that it is possible to correct any discrepancy in leg lengths, usually caused by shortening of the affected leg because the joint surface is worn away. Trial reduction is now performed to ensure that the new hip is stable and has got a good range of movement and the leg lengths are equal. If these conditions are satisfied, acrylic cement is introduced down the central cavity of the thigh bone and the stem pushed down into it. It usually takes 8 minutes for the cement to 'cure' (go hard), and after this the hip is put back into position in the socket and the muscles and skin are stitched up.

With careful positioning of the acetabular cup and using a stem of appropriate neck length it should have been possible to correct the leg length (within reasonable limits) and to correct any deformity so that the legs lie in alignment and are of equal length. Clearly where leg length discrepancy and deformity have been severe, it may not be possible completely to correct them. This would put an unacceptable stretching on the sciatic nerve which could lead to marked weakness of the lower limb. Similarly, if deformity is severe there is usually secondary contracture of the muscles and ligaments around the joint and to attempt to correct the deformity completely would necessitate

Total hip replacement: the hospital stay

dividing those tightened muscles and ligaments so that the hip would be very weak afterwards. Rarely it will be found that because of very lax capsules and muscles that the stem that would give the perfect leg length is not stable, that is, it dislocates easily, and it may be necessary to put in a longer necked stem to make the hip stable and thus marginally increase the length of the limb. Many patients can accept leg length inequality of up to 1 cm without being aware of it, and this, like all aspects of behaviour, is liable to individual variation.

When you wake up after the operation, you will probably be aware of pain from the skin and muscle incisions. Also the operation usually tends to stretch out the muscles of the limb so that the leg feels tight and aches.

Most people who have a total hip replacement say that they felt no pain whatsoever, but there are a few people who do experience pain afterwards. It would be quite unrealistic to imagine that there is no pain after any big operation but once again there is marked individual variation. Just as one of two mothers who have had a normal delivery may say that she experienced no pain whatsoever during delivery of her child and the other says that she experienced severe pain — so there can be individual reactions to the operation when the total hip replacement has been quite straightforward.

Blood accumulates in the soft tissue after the operation and tubes are inserted to allow this blood to drain into sterilized bottles at the side of the bed. These drain tubes are usually left in for 48 hours after the operation. Blood transfusions will have been given if blood loss occurred to an appreciable extent during the operation. Commonly two units of blood are given amounting to one litre, and clear fluid saline is given afterwards by drip until normal drinking is established, which usually occurs by the end of 24 hours.

The drains are removed and the drip is taken down at the end of two days, and you will be allowed to get out of bed and stand with the aid of two helpers.

BED EXERCISES PRIOR TO STANDING: FIRST TWO DAYS

Including the night before the operation, the day of the operation, and two days afterwards, you will have been in bed nearly four days. The necessary starvation prior to the anaesthetic and the delay in establishing normal fluid intake afterwards, plus the large operation, does cause a shock to the system, which is more profound in the less robust. If an Olympic athlete lay in bed for four days and suffered a severe shock to the system like a total hip replacement, he would feel groggy when he first tried to stand. Loss of muscle tone causes blood to pool in the muscles and rob the circulation, so that the movement of blood and the volume of blood in the main circulation becomes reduced.

It is important to carry out certain bed exercises to improve muscle tone. In the two weeks that you will be in bed after the operation, you will be instructed to lie on your back with your feet 12–18 inches apart.

1. *Rotation of feet to encourage calf muscle contraction*
   Looking at the great toes:
   (a) the right great toe is moved in a circular fashion clockwise;
   (b) the left great toe is moved in a circular fashion anti-clockwise.
   Repeat 20 times.
2. *Quadriceps contraction exercises*
   Looking at your kneecaps, contract quadriceps muscles on front of thigh so that the kneecap moves towards your head, at the same time this pushes the knee down into the bed causing the leg to become straight.
   Repeat 20 times.
3. *Gluteal contraction exercises*
   Squeeze the buttocks together (imagine that you want to save yourself when sitting on a narrow bicycle seat and you pull your buttock muscles together to stop it hurting you).

At the same time tighten the lower abdominal muscles and breath in deeply.

Repeat 20 times.

4. *Arm strengthening exercise*

Pull yourself up on the bar that is suspended from the chain of the monkey pole above your head. This strengthens the hands and arms in preparation for using the elbow crutches.

Repeat 10 times.

These exercises can only be attempted gently in the beginning and you will gradually increase the strength applied and the number performed during the first two post-operative days, but it is advisable to continue doing them during the whole two week period that you are in hospital after the operation, performing them at least every 15 minutes when you are in bed.

STANDING OUT OF BED: DAY 3 AFTER THE OPERATION

When the drains at the operation site and the intravenous drip have been taken down, that is when you are drinking properly, it is now safe to stand and test the joint.

The implant is firmly held in the acrylic cement so that from the beginning you should commence putting your weight on the limb.

Getting out of bed (with attendants present)

1. Move to the edge of the bed.
2. Hold the operated leg in the straight position.
3. Put your hand on the bar of the monkey pole.
4. The attendant takes hold of your feet and swings them round to the floor.
5. Slide your bottom towards the edge of the bed until

your feet touch the floor, gradually sitting up to enable the operated leg to remain straight.

6. The attendant puts her foot against your toes to hold you still.
7. Place your hands on edge of the bed and push yourself upwards.
8. The attendant holds your arms to steady you.
9. Take your weight equally on both feet; this does not hurt.
10. Stand up with feet about 12 inches apart.

After standing and getting your bearings, it is time to have a walk.

At the beginning you will have a physiotherapist and a walking assistant one on each side of you and you will be using elbow crutches to help you. It is important to have slippers that fit easily and which have non-slip soles. The best type are mules that fit well up on the instep and do not have to be squeezed on over the heels. Over the first week you will be allowed to walk twice a day and you will gradually increase the distance. In between time you will be in bed doing the bed exercises to keep the muscles in good tone.

During all of this time you will be getting stronger as the bodily systems gradually get back to normal. It is important to drink plenty during this time, at least three litres a day. Your sense of taste will be changed for three to four days and you will not feel like eating very much, but it is important to drink fluids — water, tea, fruit juice, beef tea, etc.

The first bowel action usually takes place at the end of day three. A nursing attendant will help you to use a bed pan. Occasionally opening medicines or a suppository is needed to encourage matters. It is unusual for the appetite to return until you establish satisfactory bowel actions once more.

At the end of eight days or so you are allowed to sit in a chair, but your foot must be put on a foot-stool, to prevent swelling of the ankle. During the time that you are sitting in the chair, you will continue the 'bed' exercises for calf, thigh, and buttock muscles as before, but pushing up on the arms of the chair to substitute for the monkey pole.

Your walking will take place from the chair and your attendants will give you gradually decreasing help as you get up from the chair.

Getting up from the chair

1. Ensure that your elbow crutches are to hand.
2. Push the foot-stool slightly to the side with the non-operated leg.
3. Hook the non-operated foot under the heel of the operated leg and lower it slowly to the ground.
4. Put your arms on the sides of the chair and push your bottom forwards until you are sitting on the edge of the seat — holding your operated leg straight.
5. Bend the non-operated knee so that the foot is a little under the front edge of the chair.
6. Put your hands on the front of the arms of the chair on either side.
7. Push upwards with your arms and the non-operated leg.
8. As you straighten up bring the operated foot backwards so that you are standing upright with feet about 12 inches apart.
9. Take hold of the elbow crutches one at a time.

You are now in a position to start walking.

Getting back into bed

This is of course a reversal of getting out.

1. Go up to the side of the bed using elbow crutches.
2. Place the elbow crutches in convenient position.
3. Turn round and sit on edge of the bed holding the operated leg straight out.

4. Lean backwards on the bed and use the non-operated leg to push you on to the bed.
5. Lift up and take hold of the bar of the monkey pole with one hand.
6. Push on side of the bed with the other hand.
7. Hook the foot of the non-operated leg under the heel of the operated leg and lift it upwards on to bed.
8. Swing round until both legs are on the bed.
9. You will now be lying at the side of the bed.
10. Continue to hook the non-operated foot under the other heel and pushing with one hand and pulling on the monkey pole with the other, lift yourself to your usual position in the middle of the bed.

WALKING

The elbow crutches or walking sticks are used to support the operated leg during the recovery period. Elbow crutches do give more support than walking sticks, but some people prefer sticks as they find elbow crutches difficult to manage. Walking using the elbow crutches is strongly advocated during the recovery phase as the muscles are becoming stronger. In the first four weeks they are essential to enable walking to take place, but as strength returns they may not be so important. One often hears of patients who didn't need any support from four weeks after the operation, these patients are the exception rather than the rule. If a patient attempts too rigorous activity after operation they can stretch the muscles and not regain good tone and strength so that a limp persists. In addition, in the later stages of recovery, whereas the elbow crutches may not be needed at home and on level ground with nobody liable to bump into you, if you are outside in crowds or on uneven ground, the elbow crutches give good support if you suddenly stumble and also act as warning to people not to bump into you.

There are two methods of using crutches for walking.

Total hip replacement: the hospital stay

1. Tripod gait (Fig. 17)

(a) Put your weight equally on both feet.

(b) Lift both crutches together and place them about three feet in front of you.

(c) Lift the operated foot forwards to the same level as the crutches.

(d) Push downwards on both crutches to take your body weight.

(e) Lift the non-operated leg forwards to the same level as the operated leg.

Forward movement is achieved by repeating the above. As strength and confidence returns, the next stage is reached.

2. Alternate step gait (Fig. 18)

Keep the crutches in both hands.

Make forward progress by taking a step with the operated foot and bringing the crutch on the opposite side forwards at the same time, as in marching.

Take your weight firmly on the operated leg and the opposite crutch.

Take the non-operated leg forwards, at same time swing the opposite crutch forwards.

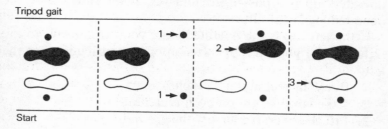

Tripod gait

Start

Fig. 17. Tripod gait. The first stages of walking: progress has to be slow because paces are very short, with the feet being brought alongside each other at every step (black foot = operated leg; black spot = crutches or stick).

Hip replacement: the facts

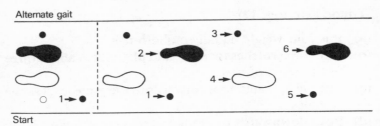

Fig. 18. Alternate step gait. This is achieved at a later stage. Walking is more natural and progression more rapid (black foot = operated leg; black spot = crutches or stick).

Forward progress with this method is clearly more rapid and natural than tripod gait.

It is important to become fully confident with alternate step gait before dispensing with one of the crutches. The first crutch to be dispensed with will be that from the same side as the operation. Normal walking, swinging the arms, is performed by bringing forward the opposite arm and this is the hand that should hold the crutch.

TURNING ROUND (FIG. 19)

You will need to be able to change direction when using the crutches and it is important not to swing your body weight round on the operated hip, that is, when turning round, the operated hip is a passenger, and you swing round with the operated leg in the air.

If the left hip is the operated side, you turn always to the right, if the right hip is operated upon you turn always to the left.

1. Put your feet about 12 inches apart.
2. Take your weight on both crutches.
3. Lift the operated leg off the ground.
4. Rotate on the forefoot of the non-operated leg to the same side — quarter turn.
5. Swing the operated leg round a quarter of a turn and put the foot down.

66

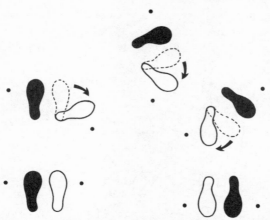

Fig. 19. Turning round (black foot = operated leg; black spot = crutches or stick).

6. Lift the crutches square to the level of the feet again.
7. Repeat a further quarter turn.

CLIMBING STAIRS (FIG. 20)

The activity is first of all performed with a helper in attendance.

The operated hip may be either the right or the left and the hand rail of the stairs may be either on the right side or the left. The stick or crutch goes into the hand opposite to the stair hand-rail.

There is a simple jingle to help in climbing stairs: 'the good leg goes up to Heaven, the bad leg goes down to Hell', where good leg refers to non-operated leg and bad leg to the operated leg.

1. Keep the crutch in one hand and hold the hand-rail with the opposite hand.
2. Push firmly down on the crutch which is on ground level and hold the hand-rail firmly.
3. Raise the non-operated foot on to the first step.
4. Push firmly on the crutch and hand-rail.

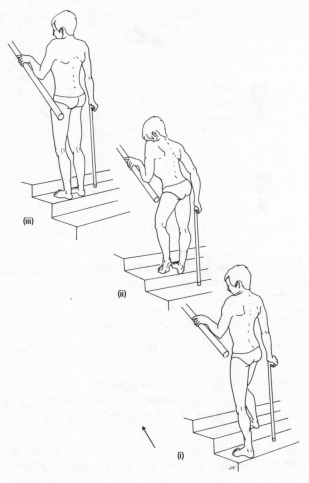

Fig. 20. Going up stairs.

5. Raise the operated leg on to the first step.
6. Taking your weight mainly on the non-operated leg raise the crutch and bring it up on to the first step.

Ascent of stairs is achieved by repeating the above sequence.

DESCENDING STAIRS (FIG. 21)

1. As before, the crutch is held in on hand and the hand-rail in the other.
2. Push firmly down on to the crutch which is at the upper level, and hold firmly to the hand-rail.
3. Lower the operated foot on to the first step going downwards.

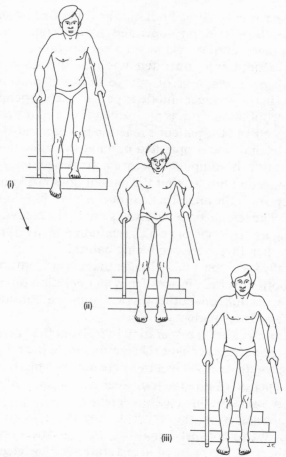

(i)

(ii)

(iii)

Fig. 21. Going down stairs.

4. Push firmly down on the crutch and hold the hand-rail firmly.
5. Lower the non-operated foot down on to the top step.
6. Taking your weight mainly on the non-operated leg lift the crutch down on to the first step downwards and slide hand down the hand-rail to reach same level.

Descent of stairs is achieved by repeating the above sequence.

In those patients where both hips are operated upon at the same time, there is no 'non-operated' leg and stair climbing is not encouraged until six weeks after the operation.

To have both hips operated upon at the same time is frequently practised, but of course it would only be contemplated in the younger and fitter patients. The operation on the most troublesome hip is performed first and if the operation goes well and the patient's reaction has been satisfactory, then the second side is operated upon at the same time. The first operation is completed before a final decision is made about the second hip, so that the patient does not know until waking up from the anaesthetic if one or both hips have been replaced. The female patients always ask in the recovery ward on waking up 'Is it one or two?', reminding many of them of the days when they were producing babies!

Generally speaking it takes longer to recover from an operation on both hips than it does from an operation on one hip, and an operation on both hips will only be considered in younger and fitter patients.

It is common after the operation to feel that the operated leg is longer than the other side. This results from the restoration of the leg length of equal length where normal length feels too long for a period of three to four weeks. As a result of gradual increase in mobility this feeling regresses.

The muscles from the pelvis to the thigh bone will be stretched out to 'proper length' if the operation on a previously short leg has resulted in restoration of leg length. This will cause a pain to pass down the front and side of the thigh with a feeling of tightness. In a similar way, with increasing mobility it is usual to find that this tight feeling, occasionally amounting to pain, gradually goes away.

If the pelvis has been hitched upwards to protect the hip before the operation, in a similar way pain can occasionally be experienced at the base of the spine or at the posterior aspect of the buttock after operation. This is usually due to stretching of the buttock muscle and can be expected to subside with increasing mobility. Occasionally, however, it is due to coincidental degenerative change in the lumbar spine that has been masked by the greater pain in the degenerate hip. This lower back pain can usually be overcome by a simple session of exercise to relax the muscle.

SIDE UNROLLING EXERCISE TO RELAX SPINAL MUSCLES (FIG. 22)

Stand with feet slightly apart, hands by the sides, and gently unroll sideways until the fingertips are level with the knee caps, pressing the hands into the side of the thighs during the whole of the exercise to unroll the spine. Move gently from

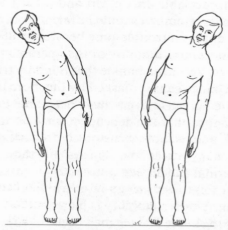

Fig. 22. Side unrolling exercise to relax spinal muscles.

Hip replacement: the facts

side to side with no stopping in the middle. Repeat 50 times to each side, each session, and carry out at least 4 sessions daily.

Whereas both hips are affected in approximately 25 per cent of people, in the remaining group with only one hip affected, it is common for up to a third of these to suffer from deterioration in the second hip one to several years later. When one hip has been causing severe pain all attention is focused on it and when the pain from that hip is relieved by joint replacement, it is frequently found, in the post-operative phase that the patient becomes aware for the first time of pain in the non-operated hip. This hip may be in an early stage of degeneration and had not previously caused symptoms. In the early post-operative phase it has more strain put on to it as it is carrying and supporting the operated limb. It is often distressing for a patient who has just gone through one big operation to feel that they are going to need a further operation before they will regain full mobility. It should be realized, however, that the extra strain imposed on the non-operated hip is a temporary situation and as the operated limb increases in strength, the extra strain will be reduced. At the end of three months it is rare for a hip with minimal change shown on the X-ray to produce any appreciable discomfort and the fear of a further operation recedes. Comfort should be taken from the fact that if the hip has not been troublesome before it will settle down quickly with increasing mobility of the operated limb.

In a similar way a knee or ankle that is mildly troubled with degenerative change can be masked by the more troublesome hip above. The patient will not have been able to do a great deal of walking, so that the dependent knee or ankle has not been stressed and is not accustomed to repeated weight-bearing. In many cases the X-rays of these joints are completely normal and all that is necessary is reassurance that the dependent joint needs to go into 'training' so that it will stop being painful after mobility is increased.

Swelling of the ankle and leg may occur as a result of interference with blood circulation from the limb. It is important to

Total hip replacement: the hospital stay

prevent blockage of the lower limb veins by keeping the lower limbs horizontal and avoid sitting in a chair with bent legs (feet on the floor). When sitting in a chair put the feet on a foot-stool and rotate the feet as indicated in the bed exercise for calf contraction.

When you can get in and out of bed, up and down from a chair, and can climb stairs and when wound healing and walking activity are deemed satisfactory it is time to go home. The hospital stay lasts from 10 to 14 days but can be longer if walking re-education is prolonged.

During the whole hospital stay you have been lying on your back in bed with the feet separated and this discipline should apply during the first nine weeks after the operation during which time the capsule of the joint is healing, the cement bone bond of the implant is maturing and the muscles are increasing in strength.

9

Return to normal function after total hip replacement

At the end of the two-week hospital stay, when the connecting activities of getting in and out of bed, rising from and sitting in a chair, and climbing stairs have been mastered, and walking using two elbow crutches comes naturally it is time to go home.

You will have had full physical support in hospital with every need being catered for, but this sort of care is not always available at home. Although you will be able to walk using the elbow crutches, you will not be able to stand for long periods, so you will also need help at home: someone to prepare meals, to help you to dress, and to ensure that everything you need is within easy reach. You will not be able to manage if you go home to an empty house and have someone calling in at odd times. If you have no close relatives and live alone, you should arrange to have further convalescence in a nursing home where the level of care is less than a hospital but more than a hotel. Often two weeks spent in a nursing home can act as a halfway house between hospital and home and smooth the transition. It is quite common for elderly patients who only have an elderly spouse at home to spend this extra time in a nursing home.

In the first six to seven weeks after going home, the elbow crutches, preferably, or sticks are used to make walking more easy. You will probably not feel like venturing out of the house in the first few days after returning home, but at least once an hour you should get up out of the chair and have a walk, gradually increasing the distance.

Your chair should be one which is not too low, a sturdy

Return to normal function after total hip replacement

dining chair with arms is ideal. When getting out of the chair you should take the precaution of moving to the edge of the chair, while keeping the operated leg as straight as possible, as described on p. 63. When sitting, you should avoid allowing the foot to rest on the floor in one position for long periods, as this causes the ankles to swell. If ankle swelling does occur towards the end of the day, it can be reduced by doing the foot circulation exercise (p. 60).

Before you were discharged from hospital you will have had a blood test to see if the operation has caused anaemia. If you do have anaemia, you will have been prescribed iron tablets and vitamin supplements. Even if you do not have anaemia it is important to eat as much fresh fruit as possible after the operation as your body needs more vitamin C after a major operation. The vitamin C you get from fruit will be more beneficial than the vitamin C you get in tablet form. Green vegetables, such as sprouts, and some drinks, such as port wine are also valuable sources of iron. Not everyone is well able to tolerate the change of diet when in hospital and they tend to regain a normal appetite only when they return home.

Hospitals can be noisy places and you may have been pre-scribed sleeping pills at night. You will of course sleep much better when you are back in your own bed, but no harm will come if sleeping pills are continued for a week or two after you return home. In hospital pain-killing pills are given to relieve the aching you feel after you first start working again. The need for pain-killers varies between patients, and some people may need to continue to take them after they return home. The judicious use of pain-killers for two to three weeks after discharge from hospital will certainly help some patients, and is harmless.

The aim of rehabilitation is to gradually increase activities to permit a full return to walking activity. The emphasis is on *gradual*: there is no need to strain until a sweat breaks out on your brow. What you want to achieve is a good strong hip at the end of a four- to six-month period that will give good function for up to 20 years — we do not want a miracle result at six weeks that will start to come loose at the end of 18 months because the cement–bone bond holding the stem has broken down. If you undertake excessive activity in the early days after the operation you may well be loosening the stem or cup. I once encountered a patient who had a total hip replacement inserted 18 months previously. His leg was gradually shortening because the stem was slipping down inside the thigh bone. He had been encouraged to ride an exercise bicycle at the end of the first week after the operation. He had made a remarkable recovery in the six months after leaving hospital but his condition had then begun to deteriorate because he had clearly overloaded the cement–bone bond and gradual loosening had occurred.

The hip needs to be kept reasonably straight and allowed to flex upwards gradually, i.e. to bend up towards the abdomen. The hip is most stable when you are in the standing position with your legs apart; it is least stable when your legs are flexed up towards the abdomen and brought across the midline. To avoid dislocation, you will be given instructions to avoid strongly flexing the hip upwards in the first six weeks after leaving hospital. In the same way you should avoid the sort of strain involved in, for example, bending forwards to tie a shoe lace or picking something off the floor with the knees straight (Fig. 23). If it is necessary to pick something off the floor when sitting down, attempt to use the helping hand device (Plate 10). If this device cannot be used, stand up and allow the operated leg to go out behind you, hold in the straight position and bend the non-operated knee so that the ground can be reached. In this position the hip is held straight and will not be in danger of dislocating.

You will be instructed to sleep on your back and avoid sleeping on your side, and told not to cross the legs in the first six weeks after going home. During this time the capsule of the hip joint is healing and with the return of muscle strength the hip will gradually become stronger. Many people are not

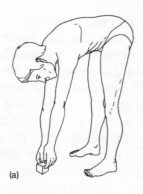

(a)

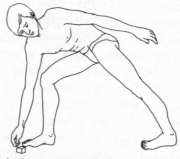

(b)

Fig. 23. Bending to touch the ground: (a) wrong and (b) right way. The left hip has been operated upon.

accustomed to sleeping on their backs, but a pillow placed between the legs helps in this respect.

Towards the end of this six-week period you will be able gradually to dispense with one crutch, and, in the house, with two if you can use furniture to gain support. The kitchen is usually the first place that this happens because most of the furniture, that is the kitchen units, is stationary, and particularly suitable to give good support because of its height and stability.

Many people ask if a bed needs to be bought downstairs for the early post-operative phase. I used to recommend this at one stage, but in the case of men I found that they usually preferred to climb the stairs to shave in the bathroom, thus defeating the object! I have tended to drop this advice. When two hips have been operated upon, however, it is a great advantage to avoid climbing stairs in the first six weeks after operation unless the patient is very fit with strong arms.

At the end of the first six weeks at home it is usually not difficult to dispense with one of the elbow crutches and to start to regain a normal walking pattern. The rate of regaining full walking function varies from patient to patient and is dependent upon the degree of muscle wasting before operation and the amount of walking afterwards. You cannot sit in a chair and expect to be able to walk normally. Similarly you must become less dependent on the elbow crutches so as to stimulate a gradual increase in muscle function. It is important always to walk as correctly as possible — take short strides, with the foot pointing forwards to begin with, walk steadily, and build up from there. Do not take large poorly controlled strides as this encourages bad walking habits, for instance some patients persist in walking with a stiff-hipped gait so that they walk 'like a clothes horse'. It is important that you be supervised by a physiotherapist or see your surgeon again at the end of six to eight weeks after the operation to ensure a smooth graduation to normal walking.

Quite often, after excellent pain relief following total hip replacement, a limp persists because of imperfect muscle re-education. The most important exercise to regain strength around the hip is the side-lifting exercise (p. 79) which will help to eradicate the limp.

SIDE LIFTING EXERCISE TO ERADICATE LIMP (PERFORMED TWO MONTHS AFTER THE OPERATION) (FIG. 24)

1. Hold the back of a dining chair and lift the operated leg first out to the side and then backwards until the muscle

Return to normal function after total hip replacement

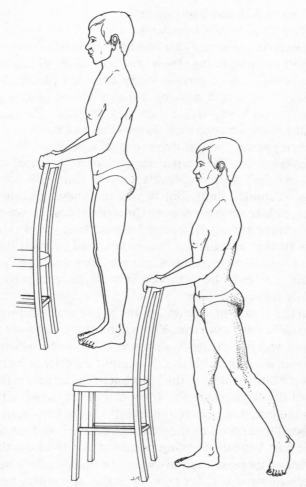

Fig. 24. Side lifting exercise.

of the buttock is felt to be tightly contracted like a ballet dancer's.

2. Hold for two seconds with the foot pointing forwards.
3. Lower the leg slowly to the neutral position (your foot will have described a triangle)

4. Repeat 30 times each session.
5. Do this at least six sessions daily.

This exercise will eradicate the limp and enable you to dispense with the remaining elbow crutch or stick. When walking outside, over uneven ground or in crowded places, it is an advantage to retain a walking aid as this will give you confidence in walking. If you go too far and feel yourself becoming tired, you can then lean on the stick more heavily on the return journey and spare your operated leg.

Recovery from the limp depends upon return of muscle power. At first you will find that you can walk for short periods without a limp, but if you try longer distances the muscles, able to cope easily with short distances, become tired, and the limp returns. As recovery progresses, you will be able to walk further and further before you find yourself limping. The aim is to be able to stand and walk for unlimited periods and this can only be achieved if walking progresses at a gradually increasing rate.

With the return of strength in the pelvic and limb muscles, general agility will improve. You will be able to attempt longer distances with increasing confidence. If you overdo things and do too much it is possible that you might experience increasing pain in the limb usually at the junction of the upper and middle thirds of the thigh where the lower end of the stem is situated. This is the junction between the relatively stiff segment of the thigh bone that contains the stem and cement, and the normal flexible part beneath. Aching occurs at this level usually as a reflection of increased activity when the bone starts to build up and become strong. It does not mean that something has gone wrong, or that something has come loose.

Aching that is due to excessive activity is always relieved by rest, and if you have overdone your walking and feel aching or pain in the limb you will be well advised to rest and you will find that the pain goes away. As a result of increase in muscle strength, when you next attempt the same walking excursion you would probably find it easier. Muscles need to be strained to stimulate them to increase in strength.

It is important in the phase of gradually increasing activity to avoid forcing the hip up into flexion to prevent dislocation. Dislocation is due to strongly flexing the hip before the capsule has had time to heal. Putting on stockings and tights, tying shoe laces, and getting up from a low chair have all been the cause of dislocation.

Attempt to keep the leg as straight as possible by favouring a high chair of dining-chair height, wear casual shoes for your recovery period that do not have laces, use a long shoe horn to ease putting on shoes, sit with the feet apart, and avoid straining the hip into flexion.

When you are able to walk with one stick at the six to eight week stage it is usually safe to start driving a car. You would be wise to start off using a medium-sized car if you are above average height to avoid forcing the hip up into flexion in the same way as you would avoid a low chair. If you choose quiet traffic conditions you will soon find that driving is quite manageable in most circumstances. Your surgeon, seeing that you can manage with one stick, will appreciate that a fair level of function has returned and will give you the written authorization to begin driving that may be required by your insurance company.

Patients can usually carry out this schedule for rehabilitation without supervision, but some patients will find the supervision of the physiotherapist essential. At Wrightington hospital patients are closely supervised by physiotherapists when in hospital and the general experience has shown us that continuous supervision is not necessary after they return home.

Being able to walk with one stick indicates a fair level of muscle control and stability of the limb, but occasionally exercise in addition to side-lifting is needed, in particular to strengthen the thigh muscles coming from the pelvis. The straight leg raising exercise (Fig. 16, p. 53) is very useful if the muscles on the front of the thigh have become thin.

Hip replacement: the facts

If walking using one stick is possible further activities can be undertaken, in particular sleeping on the side, and subsequently marital relations.

To start to sleep on the side at the end of six to eight weeks it is necessary to maintain good tension in the important pelvic muscles to keep the hip in its stable position.

Lying directly on to the operated hip may be painful at this stage as the muscle layer is still irritable. Lie on non-operated side with:

(1) pillow between thighs for one week;

(2) pillow between knees for one week;

(3) pillow between shins for one week;

then start to sleep normally.

When you are able to sleep comfortably on your side it is possible to commence marital relations.

It is important to have a firm bed so that in lying down the hip remains reasonably straight. The position of stability of the hip joint is the straight hip with the feet 12 inches or more apart. This is a common position for sexual intercourse for the female patient with her partner lying on top. It would be unpleasant however to have weight placed on to the newly operated hip and a more satisfactory position is for the female to lie on her back and her partner to lie alongside on the opposite side to the operated leg. The operated leg is moved out to the side and the non-operated leg is lifted upwards so that the partner, lying on his side can make a satisfactory entry. If for reasons of bodily dimensions, entry cannot be made from this position, it would be wise to wait a few weeks until the female can tolerate bearing her partner's weight on top of her.

In the case of the male patient, he is similarly in a position of stability when lying on his back and his partner should assume the superior position. If this is not practicable or desirable then waiting a few weeks will restore further strength and agility to enable the accustomed position to be resumed, always remembering to avoid strong flexion of the hip.

Return to normal function after total hip replacement

Increased walking leads to overall improvement in function. Some patients do not have the patience to walk long distances and they can find an exercise bicycle most useful in that it appears 'to speed things up a bit'. It is an excellent activity because muscles are stressed without the full body weight being borne on the hip joint so that straining of the muscles is rarely encountered.

Walking is good for you, jogging very bad. The sudden jolt of the limb in jogging is injurious to the cement–bone junction and is a potent source of loosening. Similarly, games that involve sudden twisting are also not to be encouraged. Whereas golf and leisurely tennis are allowed, it is not a good idea to play sports such as soccer, hockey, rugby, or squash.

The younger patient who is seeking exercise to make him pant should confine himself to cycling or swimming because here full muscle activity is performed without bearing full body weight. Some activities of cricket — slip-fielding, batting, but using a runner to run between the wickets — do enable sensible people to have the best of both worlds.

The rate of recovery varies with the individual. Do not be disheartened by the statement 'Mr Whatsisname was walking without any crutches four weeks after the operation'. Patients who rush things in the early stages can often stretch the muscles and finish up with a rolling gait.

Do keep a check on your progress — try to do more each day and note landmarks of either distances walked or time spent walking before becoming tired.

At the end of three to four months the muscles should have regained in strength and any deformity of the limb that was present before the operation should have been realigned. A leg that previously felt too long should now feel the normal length.

Occasionally it is not possible to fully correct leg length inequality and at this stage it is justifiable, if the leg still feels either long or short, to add the appropriate heel correction.

10

Total knee replacement

If you are having a total knee replacement operation your general health will be assessed in the same way as it would be if you were having the hip operation. You will undergo the same general physical checks and anaesthetic assessment, but the skin preparation will be confined to the lower limb from the groin downwards for shaving and skin sterilization. The skin and whole lower limb must be free of any infection or ulcer.

THE OPERATION

The incision curves lengthwise around the inner side of the knee joint. The capsule of the joint is cut and the muscle above the knee split through the tendon. The kneecap is folded back and the joint exposed by bending the knee to a right angle.

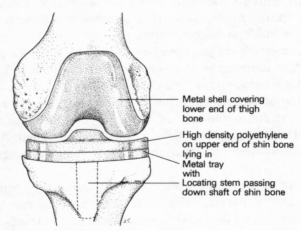

Metal shell covering lower end of thigh bone

High density polyethylene on upper end of shin bone lying in

Metal tray with

Locating stem passing down shaft of shin bone

Fig. 25. Total knee replacement.

Total knee replacement

Special tools are employed to measure the bone to indicate the level at which the bone is to be divided so as to remove the worn out joint surfaces and prepare the site for the joint replacement. The bone cuts on the thigh bone and the shin bone will be so placed as to bring the leg back into alignment if there has been deformity of either bow leg or knock knee beforehand. The knee joint has relatively flat surfaces and the replacement is fashioned to comply with these surfaces. The lower end of the thigh bone is covered with the curved prosthesis to permit the gliding, hinging movement of the normal knee with a small amount of rotation at the extreme of the range of movement.

The upper end of the shin bone has a flat plate of plastic applied to it with two gently sloped concavities in the upper surface to contain the rather flattened double balls of the thigh bone resurfacing (Fig. 25).

When both surfaces have been prepared, the trial prostheses are inserted to test for fit, stability, correction of deformity, and range of movement. If these qualities are satisfactory, it is usual at this stage to fashion the surface of the kneecap to accommodate the plastic dome replacement which will move over the lower end of the thigh bone during knee bending.

Cement is now mixed and applied to the exposed areas of bone that have been suitably prepared and the joint replacement inserted and pressed firmly into place. All excess cement is removed at the end of the operation and drains are inserted before the capsule and the skin are stitched up.

A large compression bandage is now applied. Since the knee is not covered with thick muscle, as the hip is, there would be profuse bleeding from the blood-vessels in the joint lining if compression was not applied. A back splint holds the leg in the straightened position which in the first few days after the operation prevents movement and reduces pain.

The drains are removed after 48 hours; and after four days the splint is removed. Despite the compression bandage and the drains, it is usual for a small amount of bleeding to have occurred on the dressings and the drying of the blood causes these dressings to become hard and cause discomfort. It is beneficial for the compression bandage to be taken off after four days when the back splint is removed and for the dressings to be changed, and for further support to be provided with two or three crepe bandages going from the mid-thigh to the mid-calf level.

Walking is now permitted with gentle bending of the knee, not forcing it, but allowing it to bend gently by itself. As the skin incision curves lengthwise around the kneecap, bending does not cause undue pulling on the stitches, so gently bending the knee will not cause any delay in healing.

Walking is allowed using two elbow crutches for short periods to begin with, gradually increasing from the tripod gait to alternate step gait as shown on p. 65. When you get in and out of bed or up and down from a chair, hold the leg straight in the same way as described for the hip (pp. 61, 63). However these manoeuvres are not as difficult after a knee replacement as they are after a total hip replacement.

The period in hospital need not be as long as for total hip replacement once walking has been established. The first objective is to ensure that the capsule and the skin heal properly. This is vitally important in total knee replacement because the joint is near the surface and any break in the skin could lead to infection of the joint cavity. The stitches are removed after 10–14 days.

You will spend short periods of time walking. You should spend the remaining time in bed or sitting on a chair with the leg elevated on a foot-stool. Take care to avoid standing, as this leads to congestion of the joint and superficial tissues, and to delay in the healing of the wound.

BED EXERCISES IN BACK SPLINT: FIRST FOUR DAYS

Contracting the quadriceps muscle on the front of the thigh

will cause the kneecap to move up and down in the lengthwise direction of the leg. You will not be able to see the kneecap as it will be still covered by the compression bandage, but once you are able to contract the quadriceps muscle strongly you will also be able to do straight leg raising exercises as well — these should be attempted after the first two days following operation when the drains have been removed.

Starting gently and gradually increasing in strength of contraction — the quadriceps muscle is tightened 10 times each session — and repeated hourly throughout the day.

BENDING EXERCISE

When the back splint has been removed and the compression bandage and dressings changed at the end of four days, gentle bending of the knee is permissible within the limits of discomfort. There is no hurry at this stage to increase bending, but it is often pleasurable to feel the new joint move through 20° to 30° of flexion and this gentle movement does help the soft tissue swelling to settle down. Earnest application to the improvement of bending should start only when the stitches have been taken out.

EXERCISES AFTER LEAVING HOSPITAL

Walking with the elbow crutches preferably (or walking sticks) should be continual and gradually increased. You should walk a short distance every half hour, and twice a day you should go outside the house for longer walks — keeping to well paved flat surfaces. If the surrounding thoroughfares are congested, uncrowded public parks in quiet areas are usually best.

In the same way as when recovering from a total hip replacement, even when you are feeling less need of the crutches, it is useful to continue to use them during the recovery phase for two main reasons. You will be putting less weight on the crutches when you gain increased walking ability as strength increases. You will be making greater excursions in your walking, but if you overestimate your recovery in strength and you find you have gone too far, you can put more weight on the crutches to enable you to return home.

After the stitches have been removed at the two-week stage, you should begin gradually increasing the bending of the knee, within the limits of discomfort, and you should observe a gradually increasing range of movement.

(a) To encourage knee bending

1. Sitting back in a chair with your thigh well supported, allow the shin bone to hang down and observe the bending (flexion) of the knee.
2. Lift it up to its straight (fully extended) position, hold for two seconds.
3. Repeat 20 times.

(b) To increase strength of the leg — straight leg raising (p. 53)

1. Sit forwards on a chair until your bottom is at the edge of the chair thus allowing the leg to stretch out straight with the knee in the fully straightened position.
2. Lift the foot until the leg is in a horizontal position.
3. Hold for two seconds.
4. Lower slowly.
5. Repeat 20 times.

(c) To straighten the leg

1. Sit forward in the chair until bottom is at edge of chair as in (b).
2. Place heel on foot-stool so that knee is at midpoint between the front edge of chair and the foot-stool.

Total knee replacement

3. Tighten the quadriceps to pull the kneecap up and force the knee downwards to straighten the knee.
4. Hold for two seconds.
5. Repeat 20 times.

Performing these exercises should result in a gradually increasing range of movement, however it may occasionally be necessary to increase the strength of the exercise to hurry things up.

These exercises should not be performed earlier than nine weeks after the operation as the cement is increasing in strength during this period.

Boosted knee flexion exercises

(a)
1. Sit on edge of a table with your thigh on the table but your knee completely free.
2. Place a cushion or pillow behind the knee and protecting the edge of the table.
3. Allow the leg to hang down.
4. Straighten your knee and then allow your leg to fall down under its own weight.
5. Repeat 20 times.

(b) (See Fig. 26, p. 90)
1. Place two dining chairs back to back.
2. Distance them your body width apart.
3. Place your forearms along the top of the chairs.
4. Put the operated foot forward so that the foot lies at a line joining the two front legs of the chairs.
5. Put the non-operated foot at a mid-point of the two back legs.
6. Lean forwards on to the operated knee taking some body weight on your forearm but allowing some weight to fall on your knees within the limit of discomfort, so that the knee bends.

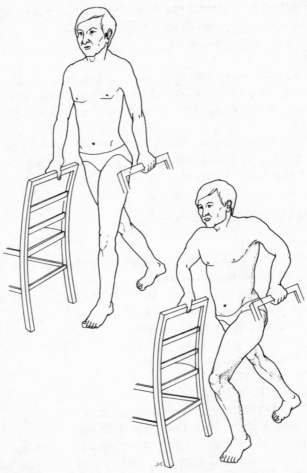

Fig. 26. Exercise between two chairs to produce greater bending of the left knee.

7. Rock backwards and forwards to increase the bending of the operated knee.
8. Gradually increase strength of the bending of the knee as you become accustomed to the exercise, by reducing weight on arms.

Total knee replacement

Boosted exercise to straighten knee (Fig. 27)

1. Stand behind chair and hold on to the back of it.
2. Push your knee forwards to bend it approximately 10° more than its fully straightened position.
3. With your body weight on the leg, snap the knee backwards now to push it into its position of maximum extension (straight).
4. Repeat 20 times gradually increasing strength of straightening snap.
5. If swelling occurs alternate with straight leg raising (p. 53).

If in spite of all these measures you still have difficulty in bending the knee, this may well be due to the development of adhesions within the joint and it may be necessary to manipulate the joint.

This does not happen very often if the above measures have been observed, but your orthopaedic surgeon will advise you about this.

The object of rehabilitation is to achieve a straight leg that will make standing comfortable and enable you to stand

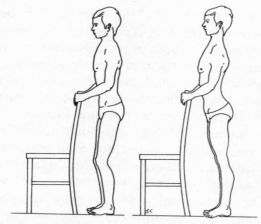

Fig. 27.   Knee straightening exercise.

upright, also to be able to bend the knee to between 90° and 110° to enable such activities as climbing stairs and getting out of chairs and out of bed to be performed easily.

Swelling of the knee can result from irritation of the synovial lining by the operation or as a result of the thickening that can be present in rheumatoid arthritis. Fluid or blood may accumulate after the operation and also lead to swelling of the joint. This joint swelling may appear large when compared to the other non-operated side as a result of weakness and wasting of the quadriceps muscle on the operated leg giving way to the bulging of the joint lining. Some swelling is quite normal as a joint reaction after operation. It will subside quickly after the operation if straight leg raising exercises are performed conscientiously. This is because when you do straight leg raising exercises, the quadriceps muscle contracts and squeezes the synovium by contracting the capsule of the knee so that joint fluid is encouraged to leave the knee joint and return to the circulation. Further support to the knee capsule to prevent congestion of the knee can be provided by a knee support such as a crepe bandage or elasticated tubular bandage. You must also remember to avoid long periods of standing.

The degenerative arthritis of the knee may have been associated with a severe deformity of either knock knee or bow leg. In the severe degrees of both of these deformities twisting of the shin bone occurs. After total knee replacement it may be observed that some twisting is still present in the shin bone. The knee replacement can only correct the joint surface and sets out, at best, to produce a horizontal joint surface which will provide long-term stability. You should not be alarmed if, after operation, your leg does not look completely straight. If the ankle is horizontal and the articulating surface of the knee replacement is horizontal also, then you can be assured of good function, even though it will not have been possible to fully correct the severe deformity.

Swelling of the ankle may occur as a result of immobiliza

Total knee replacement

tion and constriction by the compression bandage and can sometimes persist after the compression bandage has been removed. This swelling will be aggravated by standing or sitting, or lying with the knee bent over a firm edge. The foot rotation exercises (p. 60), encourage the fluid to return to the circulation.

The operation involves cutting into and stitching the capsule of the knee joint. This results in a minor amount of over-lapping of the capsule so that it is tight afterwards. This tightness of the capsule can be experienced as a general feeling of tightness of the joint when bending the knee after operation and can last up to three months. It is felt most of all at the bottom of the incision below the kneecap. As the knee begins to bend more easily the capsule gradually stretches to accommodate this movement and the feeling of tightness subsides. During this period the knee will benefit from a crepe bandage or tubular elastic support, 'Tubigrip' being particularly useful.

Three weeks after the operation the incision has usually firmed up and it is safe to have a shower or, with help, get into a bath. Inadvertently bending the knee to an excessive degree, as for example, slipping when getting out of the bath, may suddenly push the knee through a greater range of flexion and cause pain as a result of synovial lining irritation. This will result in a swelling of the joint. Rest and support will help this to settle down and a reduction of pain and swelling with rest indicates that the upset is temporary.

If the degenerative knee condition is the result of rheumatoid arthritis — occasionally there can be a sudden onset of pain and swelling in the joint as a result of an exacerbation of the generalized polyarthritis. Patients may be alarmed that something has gone wrong, the most frequent concern is that the joint may have become infected. Even though the joint surfaces have been replaced, the synovial lining is still present and it is possible for a flare-up of generalized rheumatoid arthritis to affect the synovium even in a replaced knee joint.

Hip replacement: the facts

The local pain and swelling are seldom severe and settle quickly with treatment of the generalized rheumatoid arthritis.

If the function in a normal knee is called 100 per cent, the best knee replacements are at present offering about 80 to 85 per cent of normal function — this normal function including pain relief, stability, and movement. This is to be contrasted to the total hip replacement, which being a simple universal ball and socket joint is much simpler mechanically and probably gives 90 to 95 per cent of 'normal' function. Present total knee replacements represent a gradual improvement in overall function over the last ten years, and further improvement will occur, but they have not reached the very high level of total hip replacement — which in the 60 year old can fulfil all that is required of it.

Doctors hesitate to offer total knee replacement to younger patients because they do not know how stable such replacements are over a lifetime, and how the cement–bone bond will behave over such a period. The percentages quoted above are a rough guide to function, but to gain the worthwhile overall benefit of total joint replacement, a patient with a painful knee has to be marginally worse off before the operation than a patient with a painful hip.

11

Complications

A total joint replacement is a procedure involving high technology. It is an outstandingly successful operation, but risks are involved. Travelling by aeroplane is extremely safe, but there are risks in that air crashes can occasionally occur. In the same way, there are risks with any operative procedure in that death can occur as a result of complications that are present in any operative procedure. These are: reaction to anaesthetic gases: sudden collapse from cardiovascular failure: fat embolus (a little understood phenomenon where there is a precipitation of fat in the bloodstream); pulmonary embolus, where a blood clot travels from the leg to the lungs after operation; or infection of the operative site. Stringent medical checks are made in an attempt to assess susceptibility or tendency to cardiovascular or respiratory complications during surgery. The precautions taken to avoid infection are detailed in the description of ultra clean air (p. 36).

Mobilization is rapid after total joint replacement in an attempt to reduce the dangers of blood clot travelling from the leg veins to the lungs — pulmonary embolus. If this condition is severe, it can be fatal. In a large number of patients the complications work out at roughly 0.5 per cent. It is necessary, however, for the doctor to always ensure that any given patient is sufficiently disabled by the degenerative joint condition to merit the risks that are involved in a high technology procedure, even though these risks are small.

INFECTION

If in spite of the measures that have been taken, infection

occurs at the time of operation, it is usually necessary to give a course of antibiotics to see if this can be eradicated. Fortunately this is very rare. It is more common, however, for an infection to appear some time after operation, maybe three to four years later. This can sometimes occur as a result of organisms that are present in the bloodstream settling on the joint replacement. Patients with rheumatoid arthritis appear to be more prone to this and any patient who has a joint replacement who has any existing infection at the time of the operation, be it a boil on the neck, a sore throat, or nailfold infection, should always have a course of antibiotics as a means of preventing infection of their implant. In addition, in the same way that any patient that has a heart valve replacement would always have a course of antibiotics if they were having teeth extracted, patients with total joint replacement should do likewise. It would appear that patients who are on steroid therapy for any reason, or have rheumatoid arthritis, or who are in reduced general health are prone to the development of infection and they should take special care and consult their doctor at the first sign of an infection.

LOOSENING OF THE IMPLANT

Attempts are made at the time of surgery to produce a high pressure bond in the implant. This bond distributes the load over the whole of the area of the bone to which it is fixed so as to reduce the occurrence of loosening. Loosening can occur, however, if a joint is subjected to excessive loading and this is something to be avoided. If someone has a hip or knee replacement we know from experience that it will withstand unlimited periods of walking and standing, but it will soon loosen if it is subjected to jogging. This is particularly relevant in the younger patients who are now having total joint replacement. In a similar way, a person with a total hip replacement or a total knee replacement should not indulge in contact sports or jump from heights on to the limb with the replaced joint. This

Complications

sudden jarring movement will probably exceed the strength of the cement bond and cause loosening. From time to time, however, the patient who has had a hip replacement may slip and fall and jar the joint. A single episode of this very rarely leads to loosening of an implant. There are often instances where patients have been involved in a road traffic accident and have sustained a fracture of the shaft of the thigh bone below the implant and the actual total hip replacement has not been disturbed. There are also recorded instance of injuries around the knee joint which is the site of a total knee replacement where fractures have occurred either above or below the knee replacement and this has not resulted in any loosening of the implant itself. Repetitive jarring of the implant, however, such as in jogging or contact sports does cause an increased rate of loosening. It is important to avoid soccer, badminton, and squash, but people with total hip and total knee replacements are able to play golf and gentle tennis from the baseline. Some patients do not feel that they are getting worthwhile exercise unless they are panting and perspiring. People with total joint replacement who wish to have strenuous exercise to produce this level of activity are advised to either swim or cycle.

DISLOCATION

This is when the ball at the end of the thigh bone comes out of the hip socket so that weight bearing is not possible. The replaced joint has a small diameter of articulation within the normal socket. The small diameter is known to produce less friction, and to give the most advantageous engineering qualities to allow a long period of function of the new artificial joint. This small diameter articulation, or ball and socket, can dislocate if subjected to unfavourable leverage. The position of stability of the hip joint is standing in the erect position with the feet about 12 inches apart. In this position the hip is completely stable and cannot dislocate. The reverse of this is

Hip replacement: the facts

the position where the hip is strongly flexed, i.e. bent upwards towards the abdomen and brought towards the midline. In this position the strong muscles that maintain the stability of the joint are relaxed and dislocation can occur if strong leverage is applied to the joint, i.e. if one were to bring the knee up to the chest and pull on the foot as in attempting to put on a tight slipper. Dislocation is particularly liable to occur in the period just after the operation before the hip capsule is fully healed. This is the reason for advising the patient to hold their operated leg straight when getting up from the seated position or in and out of bed, or in and out of a motorcar. If the rehabilitation exercises are carried out, dislocation is a very rare occurrence, but patients are sometimes forgetful and will perform a sudden movement which will produce a dislocation. As previously mentioned, attempting to squeeze on a tight slipper, necessitating strongly flexing the thigh up to the chest and pulling on the slipper, which produces strong leverage on the hip joint, can lead to a dislocation if carried out soon after the operation, but in a similar way if someone has had a right hip replaced and suddenly sits forwards and leans down to the right side similar strong leverage is applied to the hip joint and can lead to dislocation. If dislocation does occur the patient will be aware of it usually by the presence of pain around the joint and his inability to put weight on the limb. The hip needs to be put back into place, usually under anaesthetic, and the patient is often kept in bed for a period of 10–12 days with the legs held apart so as to allow the capsule of the joint to settle down. Dislocations can occur many years after a successful replacement as a result of a sudden injudicious movement. In an attempt to avoid these undue stresses it is wise never to sit with the knees crossed although it is quite safe to sit with the feet crossed, and when bending to the ground to allow some bending to occur at the knee as well as at the hip. Never bend to the ground with the knee held straight (p. 77). When a dislocation has occurred soon after the operation, it is a fairly straightforward measure to put it back in place, and the patient then needs to go back to the first phase in their rehabilitation: they should sleep with their feet parted for three weeks lying on their back, should avoid sleeping on the side or crossing their legs. Contraction of the thigh muscles to produce movement of the kneecaps will aid the healing of the capsule and promote the stability of the joint. The bed exercises of the hospital period should be performed for six weeks (see Chapter 8, p. 60).

Dislocation can occasionally occur long after the operation, that is after three to four years. This is more liable to occur in patients with rheumatoid arthritis where there may be low muscle tone. A patient can occasionally bend down abruptly to pick up a matchstick off the floor or a flower from the garden but without bending their knees, and this produces the severe strain in their hip resulting in dislocation. In these patients the dislocation does of course need to be put back and they require a period of sleeping on their back with their legs apart to allow healing of the capsule to occur and afterwards they should carry out a period of side lifting exercises for three months to promote stability of the joint (Chapter 9, p. 78).

Rarely, total joint replacement will be complicated by weakness of the foot following the operation. This is usually due to stretching of the sciatic nerve in hip operations or stretching of the lateral popliteal nerve in knee operations. A period of support for the resulting weakness or dropping of the foot is necessary and recovery is spontaneous, but can take several months.

Movement of the foot to encourage calf contraction is encouraged in the early post-operative period to promote the circulation of blood and venous drainage from the lower limbs (Chapter 8, p. 60). These measures will usually prevent swelling of the ankles and calf that indicates blockage of the veins in the leg. It is important to avoid passage of these blood clots to the lungs (pulmonary embolus) which can be a serious complication. If there is a particular tendency towards blood clots as evidenced by their occurrence in a previous operation, it is usual to give anticoagulants after the operation to prevent their occurrence.

12

Replacement of other joints

The success of the total hip and knee replacements led to the application of the same principles to other joints affected by degenerative arthritis.

The replacement of the shoulder, wrist, elbow, and ankle joint have all been practised.

THE SHOULDER

The shoulder is a ball and socket joint like the hip, but it has a shallow socket (glenoid) and a large ball (head of humerus) that overlaps the socket. The shoulder enjoys a great deal of mobility as a result of this shape and the control and strength of these movements is gained from the surrounding tendons which lead into the joint capsule.

Rheumatoid arthritis is the most common cause of degenerative disease of the shoulder. It affects the capsule and causes thickening and stiffening and eventually erodes the joint surface in the same way as it affects the hip and knee. Disability can be severe; the patient may be unable, for instance, to lift the hand to the mouth or to comb the hair, and feels pain even when not moving the shoulder at all.

Shoulder replacement (Fig. 28) is a reliable and worthwhile procedure producing great relief of pain. Whereas in total hip replacement the rehabilitation is based on walking and invariably proceeds smoothly with only occasional supervision by surgeon and physiotherapist, shoulder replacement does require continuous supervision to ensure that useful movement is gained. After successful rehabilitation, however, the level of function and pain relief can be of a very high order.

101

Hip replacement: the facts

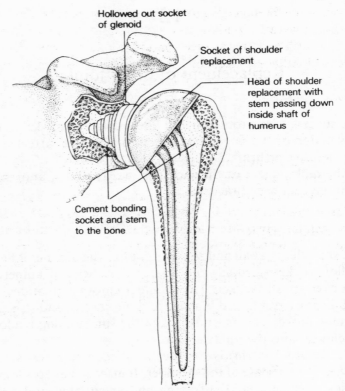

Hollowed out socket of glenoid

Socket of shoulder replacement

Head of shoulder replacement with stem passing down inside shaft of humerus

Cement bonding socket and stem to the bone

Fig. 28. Total shoulder replacement.

THE ANKLE

Arthritis of the ankle can be a part of rheumatoid arthritis or it can follow an injury. Ankle joint replacement is becoming more frequently practised but the results are not satisfactory at present compared to joint replacement in the hip and knee. It is generally conceded, even among the enthusiasts, that the results of ankle replacement for degenerative arthritis secondary to injury are poor because of stiffness. In a similar way when degenerative arthritis of the ankle occurs as part of rheumatoid arthritis, it is unusual for the joint to be affected

102

without some damage also being present in the other joints of the foot. Overall function may not be much improved as a result of residual impairment in these joints, even after a successful ankle replacement. It should be remembered that an operation to stiffen the ankle (see p. 17) can be very satisfactory in relieving pain and can allow almost a normal gait.

THE ELBOW

Elbow replacement is now gaining in popularity after a somewhat shaky start. The early joints consisted of hinges that invariably came loose. The forces passing through the elbow are of a high magnitude, higher than had originally been envisaged, and this caused loosening of the stem of the hinged implant. The newer elbow replacements attempt to mimic the design of the normal joint and there are encouraging signs for long-term stability. This procedure is still however, under study and is being performed only in special centres and will not be available in your local district general hospital for some years.

THE WRIST AND FINGER-JOINT

Wrist and finger-joint replacement has been practised now for several years and is the province of the hand surgeons. It uses silastic to form a strap on the joint, differs markedly from total joint replacement as we understand it in the large central joints, and is outside the scope of this book.

13

Special situations

The total joint replacement of the hip and knee in severe degenerative arthritis, either as a result of osteoarthritis or rheumatoid arthritis, is widely practised. A further application of the same method of treatment is its use in the reconstruction of hips following spontaneous or surgical fusion for septic infections of childhood, or the severe secondary degenerative arthritis that can occur in treated congenital dislocations of the hips. In septic arthritis of childhood, the patients are of course very young, from the age of one year up to 12 years, and since the advent of antibiotics this is now very rare in developed countries. The results of infections occurring in childhood, however, are seen in patients who are now in maturity, at the age of 50–60. In such cases the hip can be extremely stiff, with gross deformity, and in many cases the hips have fused, that is become locked. These patients will of course have a very stiff-hipped gait, with no movement at all, and they will depend on leverage through the knees and ankle joints to propel themselves forwards. They swing from side to side and rock forwards on the balls of their feet. It is very difficult for these people to negotiate stairs, or to get into or out of a chair or car. Often these patients have secondary degenerative change in the lumbar spine or the knees and this is their reason for coming forward to seek advice. They have usually found that as a result of the increased degenerative arthritis in these associated joints that their walking has often further deteriorated. Total joint replacement can restore movement to these fused hips and can result in a great increase in function. It must, however, be realized that the rate of recovery and also the amount of improvement will not be the same as a total joint replacement that was performed for straightforward osteoarthritis in maturity.

Often as a result of the septic bone condition, the normal development of the hip joint has not taken place so that there is arrested growth of the bones, the muscles, and their attachments. It is not reasonable in these cases to expect a full return to function as the muscles have not fully grown and they do not have the potential to reach normal strength. Similarly the disability has often been present for 30–40 years so that the recovery will accordingly be very slow; whereas one would expect a person in maturity with straightforward osteo-arthritis as mentioned above, to regain a reasonable level of function in four to six months, these people can take longer and often will not have reached their full potential until 18 months have passed. In congenital dislocation of the hip, the head of the thigh bone does not fit the socket properly and that is the reason that it slips out at birth or soon afterwards. The mis-match between the head of the thigh bone and the socket leads to a wear and tear which gives painful degenerative arthritis in early adult life. These patients can have a very severe secondary degenerative arthritis and come up with extremely stiff and painful hips. When this occurs with a young woman who is raising a family there are often emo-tional problems as well. It may well be that the young woman is not able to fulfil marital relations and this can lead to a strain in the marriage. These young women have a painful hip which limits their walking, they very often have young children who are demanding their attention, in addition to running a home and perhaps taking children to and from school. Whereas someone in maturity who did not have these pressing commitments would be able to accommodate to their distressing hip pain, these patients are not able to do so and frequently come up to seek advice at a younger age than the usual patient with degenerative hip disease.

Total hip replacement can produce an enormous improvement in these patients, but it must be borne in mind that the hips have not been normal to start off with and it would be unrealistic to expect the high level of function which can take place in total hip replacement in the 'normal' degenerative hip of maturity. These patients will not regain a full range of movement and their recovery of strength and walking function similarly takes up to 18 months as their muscles and bones have not been fully developed because of the long-standing hip disability.

Total hip replacement is being increasingly practised for many conditions other than the one for which it was originally intended, degenerative arthritis in maturity. Thus fracture dislocation of the hip as a result of a road traffic accident; slipping of the upper femoral growth cap which can occur in adolescence; and juvenile rheumatoid arthritis leading to severe hip disability in adolescence are all conditions that are being treated successfully with total hip replacement. These patients tend to be younger and it has brought down the average age of the patient having hip replacement. It is the success of the total hip replacement in the mature patient, the apparent 'normality' of their function afterwards, that has led to its popularity. It has now been accepted as a 'good' operation by the populace — it is a popular operation in the sense that people have accepted that if you have a bad hip you can get a new one. John Charnley is responsible for the technology that led to reliable and predictable results.

It is necessary not to adopt a mechanistic approach to total joint replacement because there are risks in the procedure and complications afterwards. Total joint replacement is a salvage procedure that should be embarked upon as a final resort. The greatest pressure for hip replacement comes from the young males injured in motor cycle accidents. They often feel that their hip can be renewed with the same facility as renewing the front wheel of their motor cycle, with a resumption of normal activities afterwards. These young men usually agree after long counselling that once the egg has been broken it is

Special situations

difficult to put the shell together again and total joint replacement is a poor substitute for their natural joint, but is satisfactory if life becomes unbearable because of deteriorated function. It often takes a period of severe disability for these young men to put their aspirations into perspective and then be prepared to accept the limitations imposed by the total joint replacement.

Total joint reconstruction should never be embarked upon purely as a means of restoring leg length. There is a limit to the amount of increase in leg length that can be achieved, and the constraint is imposed by the muscles and ligaments that pass from the pelvis to the thigh bone, and also the nerves and blood-vessels.

If severe stretching of the soft tissues takes place and the nerves and blood-verssels are damaged, the leg will be weak and the overall result disappointing.

We expect the service life of a total hip replacement to be approximately 20 years and a total knee replacement approximately 12 years. The artificial joint is intended to allow walking and standing for unlimited periods and care must be taken to avoid abuse of the joint by jogging, contact sports, or jumping from heights. When a joint becomes loose as a result of functioning for a 20 year period (in the case of the replaced hip joint) it is still possible to carry out a revision of the joint and to repair the faulty part. Whereas it is conceded that the second operation is not quite as good as the first, it still offers a high level of function. We acknowledge that after 20 years the patient is getting older and is less active and the result usually fulfils all their requirements. There is clearly a greater experience of second operations in hip surgery than in knee surgery because hip replacements have a longer history, but revision hip and knee surgery are both worthwhile procedures.

14

New developments in total joint replacement

A total hip replacement as devised by John Charnley using a stem in the thigh bone, a small diameter head, and thick socket of high density polyethylene will give good long-term function and stability for up to twenty years.

Fracture and loosening of the stem in the thigh bone occur, however, and high density polyethylene can deform under load. When high density polyethylene is subjected to high point loading, deformation occurs. If a ball bearing is placed on a flat block of high density polyethylene and a weight of 20 lb placed on the ball bearing, it will slowly deform the underlying high density polyethylene and start going down into the surface. If the ball bearing is now taken away, the hole that has been created will gradually disappear as the high density polyethylene resumes its original shape. This tendency to deform leads to an increase in frictional resistance. If the friction resistance between joint surfaces is high, then a correspondingly high stress is transmitted through the prosthesis to the cement–bone junction, which under the loads of walking can lead to the breakdown of the cement bond.

Charnley used the small diameter head to reduce the frictional resistance, but if the head diameter becomes too small it will start invaginating into the high density polyethylene.

Ceramics, in particular alumina, have been investigated in Germany and the advantages seen for this material is that it is corrosion-proof and has extreme surface hardness and wear resistance. Whereas the wear and friction of metal and high density polyethylene increase with use, the opposite happens with ceramics in that wear and friction appear to decrease with use. The difference is explained by a reduction of surface abra-

New developments in total joint replacement

sion said to result from a special bond formed between the alumina crystal and water, which provides a lubricating film between the two surfaces.

The disadvantages of ceramic is that it is brittle and when it splinters the excellent low frictional characteristic is lost.

Furthermore, in working conditions, the bone that is to receive the ceramic cup is not always of a uniform consistency in that large cysts or spaces and variations in bone structure can be present beneath the surface of the degenerate joint. It is not always possible to predict the mechanical behaviour of this bone. The fixation of the ceramic cup into this bone is often less than ideal if cement is not used. Certainly at the present time ceramics have not produced such high level results as to displace the conventional total hip replacement using metal and high density polyethylene.

The complications that are liable to arise with the hip replacement are fracture and loosening of the stem in the thigh bone. Furthermore the conventional hip replacement necessitates the removal of the head of the thigh bone and part of the neck, and if infection should occur and the implant have to be taken out, then the leg will become short.

To avoid the problem with the stem which is inserted into the thigh bone, the double cup or surface replacement operation has been developed (Fig. 29). The concept is not new, being a direct development of the Smith–Peterson single cup interpositional arthroplasty (Fig. 5, p. 20). Most double cup total hip replacements consist of a high density polyethylene acetabular cup with a large diameter and thin wall, and a metal shell round the head of the thigh bone. A stem is subjected to considerable bending forces with the metal cement–bone junction on the inner or side of the stem (a) subjected to compression while the opposite force occurs on the outer or lateral side (b) where tension or a pulling apart occurs (Fig. 11, p. 31). Acrylic cement tolerates tension poorly and the cement in this area may fragment due to the unfavourable tension forces, leading to loosening. With the double cup or femoral shell,

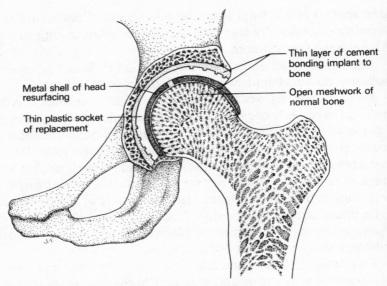

Thin layer of cement
bonding implant to
bone

Metal shell of head
resurfacing

Open meshwork of
normal bone

Thin plastic socket
of replacement

Fig. 29. Double-cup total hip replacement.

however the lever arm of the femoral neck is eliminated and
the forces are predominantly compressive (Fig. 29).

In the event of failure, an ordinary stem can be inserted
instead quite easily. In the event of infection of the double cup
prosthesis, removing the implant will leave a larger amount of
bone stock and there will be less shortening of the leg.

The increased size of the components renders this prosthesis
less liable to dislocation than the small diameter prosthesis.

So far we have only considered the advantage of the double
cup procedure, and if these theoretical advantages are found
to be valid in the clinical application of the implant, then there
would inevitably be a swing over to this procedure for the
majority of patients.

The disadvantages of the procedure are that the technique
of the operation destroys the blood supply to the head of the
thigh bone so that the bone supporting the shell may collapse.
The development of microfractures in the supporting thigh

New developments in total joint replacement

bone may be a greater potential problem, especially in rheumatoid arthritis, leading to an increased rate of collapse.

The placing of the shell may result in notching of the neck and this can lead to fracture, so that the hip becomes painful on weight-bearing once more.

The components are thinner than those of the conventional design because there is very little space between the prepared head of the thigh bone and the bed of the socket. Because these implants are advocated for the younger patient who can be expected to be more active, wear problems, especially in the plastic component, can be expected.

This operation is still under study. It cannot be advocated for all patients. The majority of total hip replacements are performed in those over 60 years old, with a high success rate when the conventional ball and socket implant is used.

The 50-year-old patient has a life expectancy of 20 years and it is thought by the enthusiasts for the double cup procedure that this operation will 'buy time', it will last for perhaps 8–10 years and can then be converted to a conventional stemmed prosthesis. However, it is recognized that first operations, with bonding of implants into fresh bone do represent the optimum conditions for producing the longest life span for a joint replacement. There is accumulating evidence now that the complications of the double cup operation are very much greater than the conventional operation. This may represent the development or teething troubles of an exciting new technique, but there is no good or convincing evidence for the widespread application of this procedure at present. The theoretical advantages of possible reduction in loosening, ease of revision or excision, and reduction of dislocation rate are outweighed by the disadvantages in practice — poor movement, poor leg length correction, loosening of cup, and fracture of neck of the thigh bone.

Further development is taking place in the fixation of hip implants in an attempt to dispense with the need for cement, even using metal stems and high density polyethylene cups.

111

Hip replacement: the facts

The surface of the stem is sintered so that the surface exhibits a fine honeycomb appearance so as to enhance the opportunity for bone to grow right up to the surface and produce good fixation. This is theoretically attractive but in the hip long-term fixation has not, as yet, been shown to be superior to stems fixed with cement.

Experimentation has also taken place with total knee replacement without the use of cement. The very high loading that occurs around the hip joint makes it unlikely that a stable prosthesis could be performed which will give good long-term stability without the use of cement. The hip joint is suited for the use of cement because the thigh bone and the socket both present concave surfaces which are ideal for compressing cement to produce high pressure bonds.

The same situation does not, however, prevail in the knee joint where the upper end of the shin bone and lower end of the thigh bone are surfaces that both do have curvatures of large diameter so that they present apparently flat surfaces for the cement–bone bond. In knee replacement it is possible to produce good long-term stability without using cement. It may well be in the future that it is possible to carry out a routine knee replacement without cement, but it is not likely with our present knowledge in the hip joint.

It is clearly important that research should continue in an attempt to improve implants and reduce the disadvantages. After all, it was dissatisfaction with the currently practised arthroplasties of the day that lead John Charnley to initiate his experiments, and thus produce his great advances.

Index

Index

Index